A NEW HISTORY OF CATARACT SURGERY

PART 3

THE HISTORY OF CATARACT EXTRACTION FROM ANTIQUITY THROUGH 1815

edited by

Christopher T. Leffler

This is the standard softcover print-on-demand edition—an accessible and budget-friendly version of this work. For those who appreciate quality, a premium hardcover edition with high-quality color illustrations is also available. Visit our website for more information.

ISBN: 978-90-6299-478-6

Wayenborgh Publishing
P.O. Box 20538
1001 NM Amsterdam, The Netherlands
www.history-ophthalmology.com

Wayenborgh Publications is an imprint of Kugler Publications, P.O. 20538, 1001 NM, Amsterdam, The Netherlands

Table of Contents

Chapter 1: Cataract Extraction from Antiquity through Daviel in 1750 . . . 1

Christopher T. Leffler, B. Frits Hogewind, Stephen G. Schwartz, Wasim A. Samara

Chapter 2: Jacques Daviel and the Presentation of Planned Cataract Extraction (1752) 65

Daniel M. Albert

1. Cataract Extraction from Antiquity through Daviel in 1750

Christopher T. Leffler, MD, MPH
B. Frits Hogewind, MD, PhD
Stephen G. Schwartz, MD, MBA
Wasim A. Samara, MD

Introduction

Cataract surgery has been performed since antiquity. The prevailing surgical technique from antiquity through much of the eighteenth century was couching, which involved pushing the opacified lens into the vitreous with a rod or needle. However, some Greco-Roman texts, and their medieval and early modern successors, seem to allude to actual removal of the cataract from the eye.

Most approaches to extracting cataracts can be classified into one of several categories: by aspirating the cataract using suction or by incising the eye and then either by grasping the cataract with instruments such as hooks or forceps or by applying external pressure on the eye with the finger.

In the case of removal of the cataract *in toto* through an incision, we demonstrate that the ancient and medieval texts are actually ambiguous and could refer to drainage of hypopyon. In the early modern period, extraction of cataracts or after-cataracts by grasping the opacity, or after creating a large incision, was occasionally discussed, even before newspaper reports of Daviel's method in 1750.

Cataract aspiration by suction probably occurred much earlier. This technique might have occurred in antiquity and certainly was performed in the medieval Arabic period. Interestingly, introduction of cataract aspiration into Western Europe could conceivably have occurred when Ottoman traveler Evliya Çelebi (1611–1682) attended peace talks with the Habsburgs at Vienna in 1665.

Overview of the Ancient Period (2nd century)

Although cataract couching was the predominant surgical technique before Daviel's work in the 18th century, cataract extraction has been discussed since antiquity. For instance, one passage of Galen in *Method of Medicine XIV* has been interpreted by Lascaratos[1] to allude to cataract extraction:

---

1 Lascaratos 1982.

> … whenever the affection is incurable, it [the best treatment] is to cut out the part together with the affection, as in the case of a cancer and all untreatable ulcers. Contrariwise, having abandoned the first indicator, as in the case of cataracts [ὑποχυμάτων, *hypochymaton*], we lead these things to another, less important place. Some [doctors], however, also attempt to evacuate these things, as I shall speak of in the [writings] on surgery.[2]

Galen does not relate here how the extraction would be performed. The methods of extraction are specified by the ancient surgeon Antyllus who indicated that one could use either (1) an inferior corneal incision or (2) aspiration by suction. Antyllus' teachings regarding cataract surgery were preserved by Abu Bakr Muhammad Ibn Zakariya al-Razi (known in Latin as Rhazes, c. 865–925) in his encyclopedia *Kitab al-Hawi fi al-tibb*, known in translation as *Liber Continens*. Meyerhof translated from the Arabic of the Escorial manuscript as well as a manuscript in his private collection:

> Antyllus says: Certain doctors have made an incision in the lower part of the pupil (cornea) [*pupilla*] and extracted the cataract [*extraxerunt catarractam*]. He continues: That is good in cases of thin (soft) cataract, but not in cases of thick (hard) cataract, because the albuminoid humour (aqueous humour and vitreous body) escape. Others have introduced a glass tube [*anbûb zugâg*] by the paracentesis opening and have proceeded by aspiration, drawing in the cataract with the albuminoid humour [*albugineus*].[3]

Ancient and Medieval Incisions: For Cataract or for Hypopyon? (2nd century)

We discuss cataract extraction by an inferior corneal incision here. Note that neither Antyllus nor Galen suggests that he has seen cataract extraction successfully performed. In addition, it is hard to be sure about the condition being treated. In the ancient and medieval periods, cataract couching was believed to displace a concretion forming anterior to the lens. Thus, occasional discussions of removing a fluid cataract by an inferior corneal incision might actually have been cases of hypopyon drainage. Indeed, in *Method of Medicine XIV*, Galen did describe drainage of hypopyon by an inferior corneal incision:

> Often, I evacuated the pus all together, having divided the external coat of the eye just above the tunic at the place where all the tunics grow together with each other. Some call the place the "iris", others the "crown."[4]

In Galen's works, the iris or crown of the eye was the limbus.[5]

---

2 Galen 2011, LCL #518, p. 487. Kühn 10.987.

3 'Ammār, Meyerhof 1937, p. 52. The Latin is from: Rhazes 1529, Book 2, capitulum 3, section QQ, car. 41, image 102. Arabic transliteration from Meyerhof 1932, p. 118.

4 Galen 2011, p. 536. LCL #518. Kühn 10.1020.

5 Leffler "medieval fallacy" 2016.

Proponents of the notion that cataract extraction was attempted in antiquity would argue that Galen and Antyllus knew the difference clinically between hypopyon and *hypochyma* (even if they did not understand a *hypochyma* to be an opacity of the lens). On the other hand, with the universally high level of misunderstanding regarding *hypochyma* pathophysiology in the ancient and medieval worlds, it is difficult to exclude the possibility that the unidentified doctors who attempted the procedure were actually draining a hypopyon. Hirschberg wrote: "Did the Greeks confuse a cataract with pus, *hypochyma* with hypopyon? Probably only those with an insufficient medical knowledge."[6] And so we are left to wonder if the unidentified surgeons who attempted to extract the *hypochyma* were more like Galen, or whether they had "insufficient medical knowledge."

Medieval oculists restricted themselves to repeating the line about extraction from Antyllus. For instance, Abu Ali al-Husain ibn Sina (Avicenna, c. 980–1037) wrote:

> Some eye surgeons have their own way. They cut underneath the cornea and have the water drip out, but this is dangerous because if the water is thicker than it is supposed to be, it will bring out the moisture of the aqueous humor with itself.[7]

We know from the early era of cataract extraction that sometimes when the inferior corneal cut was made, the unanesthetized patient would squeeze the eye shut so hard that the lens would spontaneously be expressed from the eye.[8] However, this occurrence was exceptional. Typically, the surgeon had to either make a capsulorrhexis (for extracapsular extraction) or impale the lens or apply external pressure to the eye (for intracapsular extraction). However, as we outlined earlier, the brief ancient and medieval allusions to cataract extraction by a limbal corneal incision do not mention these extra steps required to actually extract the cataract from the eye. This lack of detail argues in favor of these actually referring to hypopyon drainage.

Even when a cataract happened to accidentally dislocate into the anterior chamber during couching, the medieval Arabic oculists did not attempt to extract it. For instance, Ammar of Cairo couched a 20-year-old man from Persia with bilateral cataracts. With the left eye, "the cataract had emerged from the pupil, lay opposite to the cornea and stuck there between the cornea and the outer surface of the iris."[9] Rather than extracting the cataract with an inferior corneal incision, Ammar simply dressed the eye and found on the third day that the cataract had disappeared and the man had an acceptable visual outcome.[10]

In the 13th century, an oculist of Aleppo named Khalifah Al-Halabi asked a patient being couched to breathe in deeply to help the cataract remain depressed. The case

---

6 Hirschberg & Blodi 1985, vol. 2, p. 289.

7 Ibn Sina 2014, p. 274.

8 Leffler "Anglo-America" 2015.

9 Blodi 1993, p. 156.

10 Blodi 1993, p. 157.

was complicated for 40 days postoperatively by dislocation of the cataract into the anterior chamber. However, Khalifah's detailed case report does not end with him extracting the cataract. In fact, Khalifah was apparently satisfied with the outcome because as the cataract floated "like mercury" between the cornea and the iris, the patient still had vision.[11]

Ancient Cataract Aspiration (2nd Century)

We live in an era of cataract aspiration, but attempts to aspirate cataracts might have begun in antiquity. As noted earlier, Antyllus wrote that some surgeons aspirated cataracts through a glass tube. One can always question whether ideas only found in medieval translations might have misattributed a concept to the ancients. In fact, the works of al-Razi (Rhazes) are difficult to interpret because it is not always clear where a quotation from the ancients ends and al-Razi's own parenthetical additions begin. However, the Greco-Romans were better known for glass working than the Arabs were, and so the use of glass for the aspiration tube might suggest a truly ancient origin for the practice. On the other hand, elsewhere in this volume, Mathias Witt assembles all of the Antyllus fragments and demonstrates that cataract extraction by suction is never explicitly identified with Antyllus, and raises the possibility that this technique was not known until the medieval Arabic period.

 Max Meyerhof and other scholars have placed Antyllus in Alexandria, though another biographer guessed that he could have spent time in Rome.[12]

 Several finely crafted hollow metal needles, potentially suitable for cataract surgery, have been found at Montbellet, France, dating from about 100 CE (Fig. 1), and at Villa dels Tolegassos, Viladamat, Girona, Spain, dating from about 200 CE.[13] If these needles were indeed used for cataract aspiration, as scholars have generally believed, then the practice was established in Western Europe in antiquity. It should be noted that acceptance that these tools were used for cataract aspiration is not universal,[14] and more work could be done to explore alternate hypotheses for their use. One difficulty is that the inner diameter of the hollow needle is slightly more than 1 mm, and it would be difficult to generate enough suction to aspirate significant amounts of a senile cataract.[15] In any event, these tools demonstrate an astonishing level of craftsmanship among the Roman civilization.

---

11 Blodi 1993, p. 219–20.

12 Leffler "Annals" 2020.

13 Feugère et al. 1985; Pérez-Cambrodí 2015.

14 Savage-Smith 2022.

15 Savage-Smith 2022.

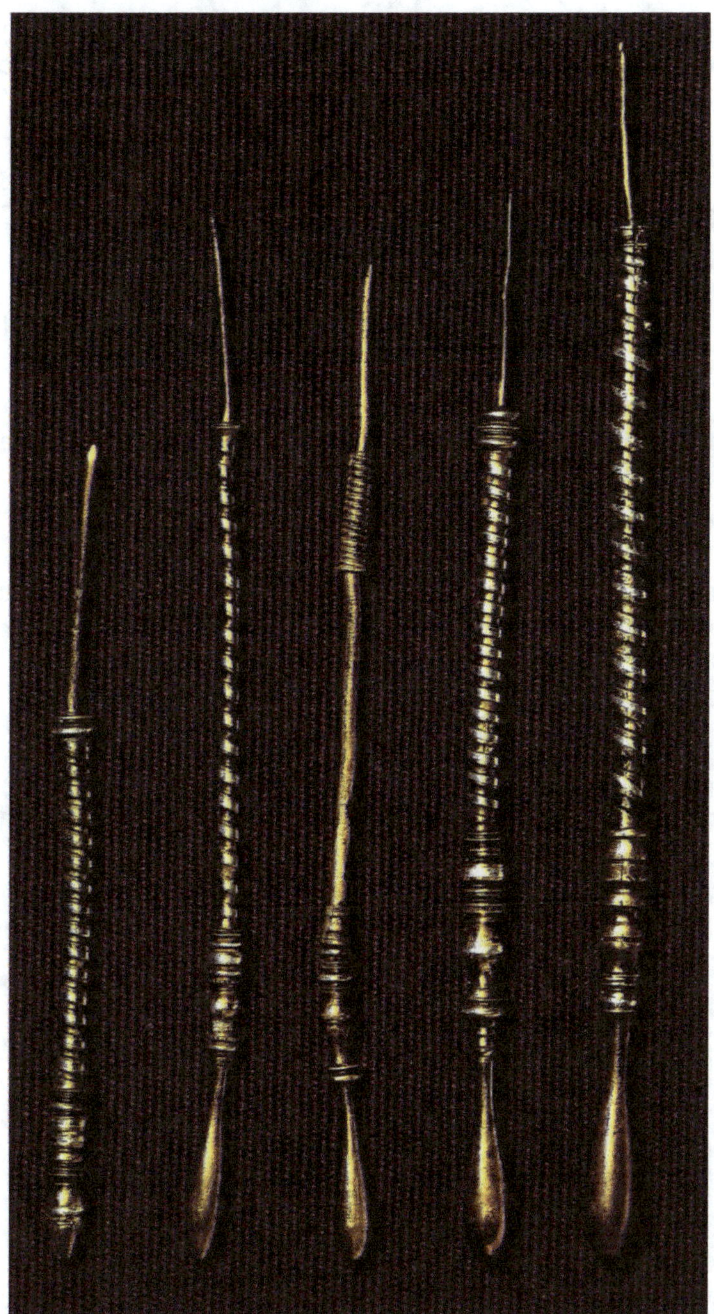

Fig. 1. Solid (numbers 1, at left, 2, and 4) and hollow (numbers 3 and 5, at right) cataract needles found at Montbellet, France, dating from 100 CE.

That the Persian author Zarrin-Dast (Goldhand) in 1087/8 CE would attribute cataract surgery with the hollow needle to the Greeks and Romans[16] is consistent with original attribution of the method to Antyllus.

Cataract Aspiration in the Medieval Arabic Period (10th Century)

As noted earlier, Rhazes in the 9th century transmitted Antyllus' description of cataract aspiration. Albucasis of 10th century Andalusia wrote:

> I have heard that a certain Iraqi has said that in Iraq he makes a hollow needle by which the humour is sucked out. In our land, I have never seen anyone do it in this fashion ...[17]

The medieval oculist 'Ammār ibn 'Alī Mawṣilī, of Mosul, who practiced in Cairo in the early 11th century, manufactured a hollow needle for cataract aspiration. He recounted that he used it first on a Christian in Tiberias:

> ... I have imagined and manufactured a hollow cataract needle (*miqdah mujawwaf*), but I did not make use of it until my sojourn at Tiberias, where a Christian took me for an operation. He said to me: Do with me what you will; but I cannot remain lying on my back! So I operated on him with the hollow needle and extracted his cataract. He saw immediately and could rest how he liked, after having dressed his eye for only seven days. No one practiced the operation for cataract with the aid of this needle before me. I have operated with it on a number of patients in Cairo and elsewhere, and they have recovered their sight. I am now going to describe it to you, as well as the way of using it, and to explain to you the reason for its triangular shape.[18]

Ammar described the hollow needle and its use as follows:

> The hollow must have the same shape as the solid needle, except that it must be thicker. The cavity must traverse it from one end to the other. The cataract is drawn into a hole pierced on one of its triangular faces. May it please Allah! That he who operates with this instrument may have need of an adroit and experienced assistant.
>
> The first moment of introduction of the needle into the eye is the same as for the solid needle. The difference in manipulation begins when the needle, introduced

---

16 Hirschberg & Blodi 1985, vol. 2, p. 71.

17 Albucasis et al. 1973, p. 256.

18 Ammar, Meyerhof 1937, pp. 47–8. In one manuscript, the case was at Baghdad rather than Tiberias (in Israel).

into the eye, has begun to couch the cataract in the same way as the solid needle. When the cataract has been couched and half of the pupil has become visible (*i.e.* black), you see the needle in the eye—look well to see on which of the three faces of the instrument is the opening, which you fit over the cataract. Then order the assistant to suck strongly; the cataract, which has a thick body (as a result of the vacuum produced by the suction) remains suspended at the opening of the needle. If that happens, bid him suck hard, while watching the cataract carefully. When the cataract has reached the hollow of the needle, remove it while the assistant continues suction without ceasing until you have removed the needle, with the cataract, from the eye. After that the patient has no needle to remain lying down; but his eye must be bandaged until the closing of the place of the paracentesis. The doctor must recommend the assistant to take care during suction that none of his breath enters the eye, which would bring about its protrusion. The doctor must also take care not to allow the needle to penetrate the albuminoid humor [aqueous humor, here also the vitreous body], which would be drawn in during the suction, causing atrophy of the eye.

After the operation the patient must avoid natural or artificial light for 40 days. He must avoid coitus, vomiting, shouting and constipation.[19]

Many Arabic authors were aware of the operation to aspirate cataracts. The hollow needle was illustrated in the treatise of Khalifah Al-Halabi of Aleppo in 1266 CE (Fig. 2).[20] Ammar's development of the hollow cataract needle was later recounted by Ṣalāḥ al-Dīn al-Kaḥḥāl of Syria in the 13th century.[21] Ṣalāḥ al-Dīn explained that Thābit Ibn Qurrah disapproved of the operation with the hollow needle on the grounds that the cataract was covered with a capsule, which was hard to penetrate, and that the healthy fluid of the eye would also be aspirated.[22] Ṣalāḥ al-Dīn thought a bronze tube would work better than the glass tube recommended by Antyllus.[23] Ibn al-Nafis was a contemporary who refined the cataract aspiration technique in Syria and Egypt.[24]

The 14th-century Egyptian oculist Sadaqah ibn Ibrahim al-Shadhili described in his treatise seeing in the market hollow cataract needles, which were supposed to work either by oral suction or by turning a screw. He was skeptical of their efficacy for a variety of reasons. Al-Shadhili lived in Cairo but also visited Jerusalem.[25] Al-Shadhili had heard of the hollow cataract needle being in the

---

19 Ammar, Meyerhof 1937, pp. 48–9.

20 Hirschberg & Blodi 1985, vol. 2, p. 201–6.

21 Blodi 1993, p. 300.

22 Blodi 1993, p. 301.

23 Blodi 1993, p. 302.

24 Pérez-Cambrodí 2015.

25 Savage-Smith 2022. Shadhili's treatise is entitled The Ophthalmological Principle in Diseases of the Visual System (*Ṣadaqa ibn Ibrāhīm al-Shādhilī in his Kitāb al'Umda al-kuḥlīya*

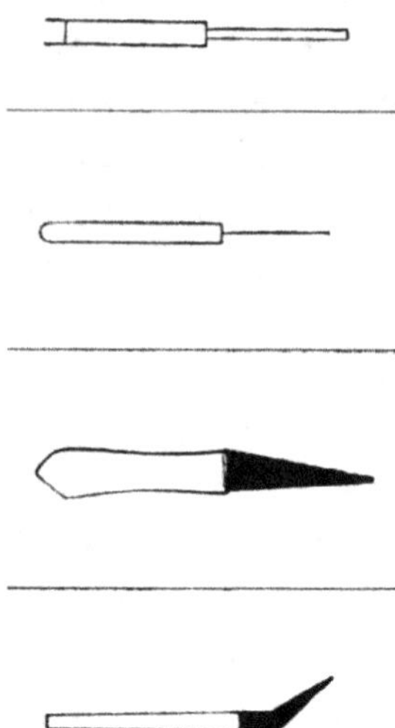

Fig. 2. Ophthalmic instruments in Khalifah's treatise (1266 CE), as illustrated in the Parisian manuscript (1273 CE). Khalifah described: (top): "Hollow cataract needle (mihatt mujawwaf). To aspirate a cataract. This operation is well known, but God knows it best." (2nd from top): "The round cataract needle (*mihatt mudawwar*) … It can be interchanged with the triangular needle [not pictured]." (2nd from bottom): "a thorn knife (*sikkīn*). With this instrument we incise the frontal arteries." (bottom): "A small knife for the sty (*dhāt al-shu ʿirah*). A lancet, the length of the blade is that of a corn of barley; also used to incise the conjunctiva for a cataract operation."[26]

instrument set of a Russian in the Roman Empire who acquired it from a Turkmen who died in his land. At that time, the Roman (Byzantine) empire would have included much of Anatolia. The closest area occupied by the "Rus" might have been the Black Sea coast in the area of the Kingdom of Galicia–Volhynia, also known as Korolivstvo Rus, or a successor state, close to the modern city of Odesa. Here is our translation from the Arabic of his account:

> When it comes to couching with the hollow needle (*Al-Maht Al-Mujawaf*), I have never used it or seen anyone else using it.[27] It is only mentioned in the books. I have seen two types of the needle ("*Al-Maht Al-Mujawaf*") and when I saw it I knew it would not work for reasons I will explain later. The first type is hollow from the tip to the head and on its side there is a tube that is used for suction by the coucher or his assistant.[28] The second type is similar but in addition has a screw (*lawlab*) on

---

26 Hirschberg & Blodi 1985, vol. 2, p. 201–6.

27 Shadhili uses the term *qadh* to refer to a cataract (Savage-Smith 2022).

28 Savage-Smith had access not only to the National Library of Medicine manuscript at Bethesda but also to the manuscript at Munich: Bayerische Staatsbibliothek, cod. Arab. 834, folios 78a-79b. She has the following in her translation: "I wish I knew whether it is the one performing the operation with the needle who does the aspirating or whether it is the surgeon's assistant who does it. Nor do I know which of them observes the cataract for his colleague as it is removed from the eye." (Savage-Smith 2022)

top that if rotated will induce suction instead of oral suction. I have tried the second type on plain water and it sucked a little bit of it. When I tried it on water thickened with mucous it did not suck anything at all. This illustrates that it would not work on the cataracts as they are thicker.

I have spoken to someone who used the second type. He said he rotated the screw and nothing came out and he had to use "*Al-Maht Al-Mujawaf*" as a regular couching needle and he hit the cataract three times with it but that patient ended up not seeing. I have asked couchers who used it and they think that maybe there is another "*Al-Maht Al-Mujawaf*" with a different design that works somewhere or maybe we are not using it correctly. It is one of those things that is written in the books and it is just there but not done in real life.[29]

Regarding the reasons why I think it will not work:

1. The diameter of the "*Al-Maht Al-Mujawaf*" is narrow and probably won't allow the cataract to be sucked. Also, if the water touches the copper it will rust after a few days and occlude the needle. You will have to use a new needle for each patient. It probably should be made from silver.
2. It is hard for the coucher [*qaddāḥ*] to tell how much he should suck out unless his assistant that opens the eye will suck the cataract out, but still it is hard to tell how much to suck which could lead to many problems.
3. If the breath of the person aspirating the cataract goes into the eye that will be a disaster for that eye.
4. The cataract is thick, so you will need someone with large lung capacity to aspirate and probably you will end up sucking not just the cataract but the other humidities of the eye and the eye will shrink.

---

29 The translation of Savage-Smith adds here: "We are thus compelled to conclude that removing the cataract [*qadḥ*] with such an instrument means either the hollow cataract needle was different in design and consequently no one [today] knows how to use it, or that in former times there were people who knew how to use it because they had seen others use it and imitated them. There are many written accounts in books of various procedures that cannot be performed nowadays because there is no one who has actually seen them performed — for example, the instrument designed to cut up a dead foetus in the womb in order to save the mother's life. Many such examples are recorded in books, but in our own time we have never seen anyone perform them because the practical knowledge has been lost, and nothing remains but the written accounts. I once got together with a celebrated surgeon (*'amāl*) by the name of Yūsuf ibn al-Labbān, who had travelled extensively, and I discussed the matter at length with him. He told me that he had made the acquaintance of numerous surgeons and had observed that some of them had the hollow cataract needle in their possession. He [Yūsuf ibn al-Labbān] said: I never saw any of them actually use it. I used to ask them to demonstrate to me how the operation was performed, but to a man they declined on the grounds that they had never seen it performed either. They said, «We have used the needle experimentally (*tajriba*) and for investigation (*mubāḥatha*), but our operations were not successful because of our ignorance of the procedure with it». [al-Shādhilī continues]: Perhaps in the past there may in fact have been surgeons who performed the operation with it [the hollow cataract-needle], but God knows best." (Savage-Smith 2022).

5. It will require a lot of experience and training before somebody is able to use it correctly, and probably there will be a lot of complications before he is able to use it safely.

6. If it worked there will be a lot of issues with aspirating too much or too little and from the breath going into the eye.

7. As far as I know the cataract is between the cornea and the pupil and when you put *"Al-Maht Al-Mujawaf"* in that space, because it has a narrow diameter, it won't aspirate the cataract and you will have to apply pressure which will squeeze the iris and the cataract will get away from your needle and you might only be able to extract some of it.[30]

8. If it had to work, it must have a bigger diameter to ease the aspiration process but at the same time it would be hard to introduce in the eye because of its bigger size.

9. I think probably for cataracts that were very dense somebody came up with this and felt very proud of it although it did not work. He just proceeded with it without explaining to others its problems.

10. I have never seen it used. It is just something out there. People hear about it, but never see it being done.

One of my friends told me that he saw a Christian Russian man in the Roman empire with *"Al-Maht Al-Mujawaf"* made of red copper and with a curved tip made of gold.[31] He asked him if he uses it. He said not really, because it is rarely successful. My friend asked him "Why did you make it then?" He [the Russian man] said he did not make it but acquired it from a Turkmen man who died in their land [the land of the Rus]. My friend asked him if he saw the Turkmen man using it. The Russian man said the Turkmen man did not use it but the Turkmen man used the regular couching needle [*al-mihatt al-muthallath al-mu'tād*] and kept *"Al-Maht Al-Mujawaf"* [the hollow needle] in front of him with his other tools. My friend asked the Russian man if he ever tried it. The Russian man said yes, he [the Russian man] did it out of curiosity, but he was not knowledgeable when it comes to using it. He [Shadhili's friend] also asked if it was ever successful. He [the Russian man] said no, and found it would loosen the cataract and might make it denser and no longer suitable for regular couching. He mentioned that he tried it on a woman and it loosened her cataract but made it denser. She did not see for a while after that but recovered some sight later.

---

30 Terms used were, cornea, *al-ṭabaqa al-qurnīya*, "hornlike tunic"; and pupil, *thaqb al-ḥijāb al-'inabī*, "the hole of the uveal membrane" (Savage-Smith 2022).

31 According to Savage-Smith, the friend described this as occurring "in the country of the Rūs [*bilād al-Rus*, north of the Black and Caspian Seas], which lies somewhere in the Byzantine lands" (Savage-Smith 2022).

> Mansur in his diary has mentioned that some people also used a glass tube with the needle but ended up sucking the white humidity (aqueous humor, *al-ruṭūba al-bayḍīya*)."[32]

Given Shadhili's overall skepticism about the ability of the procedure to succeed, some have questioned whether the procedure actually occurred, or whether it was just a "myth."[33] Perhaps, one way to think of this is as "couching-plus." Couching of cataracts has long been an option. There were times in the early 1800s when breaking up a cataract (discission) was commonly performed. Perhaps, the hollow cataract needles simply offered one additional option. The cataract could be displaced (couched), broken up, and some soft bits of cortex could on occasion be aspirated. This idea seems to correspond with Shadhili's mention of a cataract getting denser—the fluffy cortex was aspirated, but the dense nucleus remained. To the extent that some younger adults or children had soft cataracts, larger amounts of the cataract might be aspirated.

Early Mentions of Cataract Aspiration in Western Europe (12th Century)

The ancient and medieval Arabic descriptions of the technique do not seem to have had a large impact on Western Europe. Rhazes' *Continens*, which incorporated Antyllus' brief mention of the aspiration technique, was translated into Latin by Gerard of Cremona in the 12th century.[34] Gerard also translated the treatise of Albucasis, which briefly mentioned that he had never seen cataract aspiration. Likewise, Ammar's treatise, which described his aspiration technique, was translated into Hebrew by Nathan ben Eliezer ha-Me'ati in the 13th century (but never into Latin).[35] In his description of cataract surgery, Guy de Chauliac wrote in 1363:

> Some of the ancient Greeks (as Albucasis and Avicenna recite) made a hole under the cornea, with a cannulated needle pulled it [the cataract] by sucking: which I do not praise, because perhaps with the water [*i.e.* the cataract] the albugineous humor would come out: and the last error would be worse than the first.[36]

---

32 Shadhili, fol. 118a-120b. The identity of Manṣūr is unknown. Savage-Smith adds here: "And I [al-Shadhilī ?] have heard of a skilful surgeon who operated successfully on the eye of a woman of high rank while she was lying on her back" (Savage-Smith 2022).

33 Savage-Smith 2000, p. 307.

34 Compier 2012.

35 Savage-Smith 2008.

36 Chauliac 1890, p. 489.

Note that Chauliac does not indicate that he has actually seen the maneuver attempted. He cites "Rhasis" elsewhere[37] but does not mention him in the context of cataract aspiration, even though it was Rhazes who credited the Greek Antyllus with describing the practice. In addition, Chauliac wrote that Avicenna mentioned cataract aspiration, when Avicenna actually merely mentioned making an incision to drain the cataract. Finally, Chauliac does not acknowledge that the medieval Arabs were actually attempting this procedure, even though Albucasis had stated that. Nowhere does Chauliac cite the Hebrew translation of Ammar, or even seem to be aware of Ammar's work.

Galeazzo di Santa Sofia (d. 1427) of Padua described cataract aspiration by suction through a golden needle. He wrote that he had not seen that technique performed, but he included it because it seemed to him to be possible to perform.[38]

Guillaume Rondelet (1507–1566), a naturalist and sometime general physician of Montpellier, described a technique of cataract aspiration by having an assistant apply suction to a syringe.[39] Rondelet's sources are not known, and as a general physician and naturalist, it is doubtful that he would have personally performed cataract surgery.

Durante Scacchi (1596)

In the early modern period in Europe, we begin to see descriptions of cataract extraction by pulling the cataract from the eye with a surgical instrument, such as a hook or forceps. Durante Scacchi of Preci wrote in 1596 in his *Subsidium medicinae* that others had referred to removing cataracts from the eye by penetrating the eye with a hollow needle, creating a hook by bending the tip of a harp string (*citharae cordula*), inserting the hook through the hollow needle, and using the hook to extract the cataract (Fig. 3). However, Scacchi reported that he tried this surgery in animals, and it simply brought out the albugineous (aqueous) humor and tore the tunics of the eye.[40] Scacchi said he got the idea from others. Scacchi had trained with the anatomist Realdo Colombo, who briefly referred in 1559 to cataracts (*suffusiones fiunt, quas cataractas recentiores appellant*), but did not mention this technique.[41]

---

37 Chauliac 1890, p. 486.
38 Truc 1907, p. 168–9.
39 Truc 1907, p. 168
40 Scacchi 1596, p. 54.
41 Colombo 1559, p. 219.

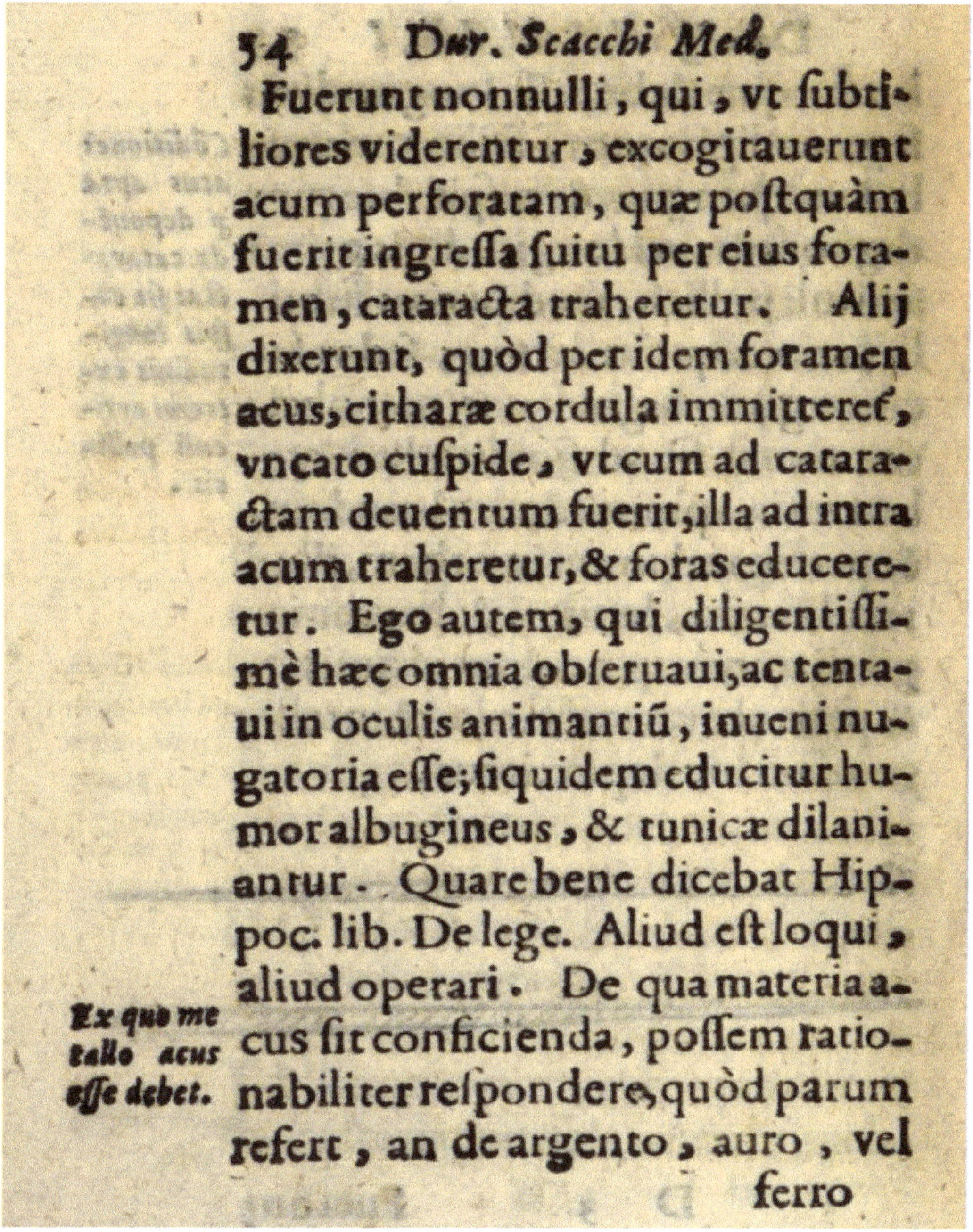

54   *Dur. Scacchi Med.*

Fuerunt nonnulli, qui, vt fubti-
liores viderentur, excogitauerunt
acum perforatam, quæ poftquàm
fuerit ingreffa fuitu per eius foramen, cataracta traheretur.   Alij
dixerunt, quòd per idem foramen
acus, citharæ cordula immitteref,
vncato cufpide, vt cum ad cataractam deuentum fuerit, illa ad intra
acum traheretur, & foras educere-
tur.   Ego autem, qui diligentiffi-
mè hæc omnia obferuaui, ac tenta-
ui in oculis animantiũ, inueni nugatoria effe; fiquidem educitur humor albugineus, & tunicæ dilani-
antur.   Quare bene dicebat Hip-
poc. lib. De lege. Aliud eft loqui,
aliud operari.   De qua materia a-
Ex quo me- cus fit conficienda, poffem ratio-
tallo acus nabiliter refpondere, quòd parum
effe debet. refert, an de argento, auro, vel
ferro

Fig. 3. Durante Scacchi discussion of cataract extraction using a hook in 1596 in *Subsidium medicinae.*

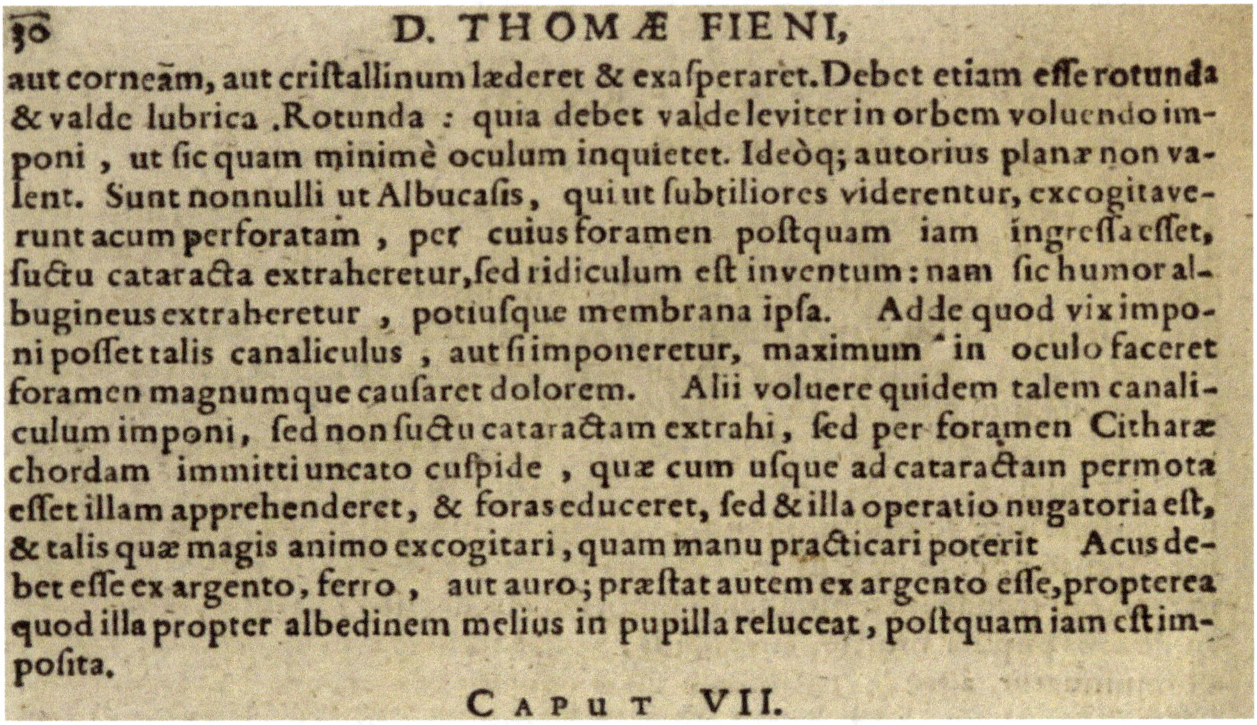

30

D. THOMÆ FIENI,

aut corneam, aut criſtallinum læderet & exaſperaret. Debet etiam eſſe rotunda & valde lubrica . Rotunda : quia debet valde leviter in orbem voluendo imponi , ut ſic quam minimè oculum inquietet. Ideòq; autorius planæ non valent. Sunt nonnulli ut Albucaſis , qui ut ſubtiliores viderentur, excogitaverunt acum perforatam , per cuius foramen poſtquam iam ingreſſa eſſet, ſuctu cataracta extraheretur, ſed ridiculum eſt inventum : nam ſic humor albugineus extraheretur , potiuſque membrana ipſa. Adde quod vix imponi poſſet talis canaliculus , aut ſi imponeretur, maximum in oculo faceret foramen magnumque cauſaret dolorem. Alii voluere quidem talem caniculum imponi, ſed non ſuctu cataractam extrahi, ſed per foramen Citharæ chordam immitti uncato cuſpide , quæ cum uſque ad cataractam permota eſſet illam apprehenderet, & foras educeret, ſed & illa operatio nugatoria eſt, & talis quæ magis animo excogitari, quam manu practicari poterit Acus debet eſſe ex argento, ferro , aut auro ; præſtat autem ex argento eſſe, propterea quod illa propter albedinem melius in pupilla reluceat, poſtquam iam eſt impoſita.

CAPUT VII.

Fig. 4. Thomas Feyens 1602 description of cataract extraction with a bent harp string forming a hook, passed through a hollow needle, and used to pull on the cataract.

Thomas Feyens (1602)

Next, surgeon Thomas Feyens (or Fienus, 1567–1631) of Louvain (Leuven) mentioned this technique in 1602 in his treatise published at Frankfurt (Fig. 4). Feyens had studied with Pieter van Foreest, Rembert Dodoens, and Girolamo Mercuriale of Italy. Feyens cited by name the Arabic author Albucasis with respect to cataract extraction by aspiration through a hollow tube. But Feyens added that one could in principle use a bent harp string (*citharae chordum*) to pull the cataract out of the eye. Feyens was skeptical of both techniques: He thought extraction by aspiration would make too large a hole in the eye and that extraction by pulling was more theoretical than practical.[42]

Both Lorenz Heister and historian Julius Hirschberg cited both Scacchi and Feyens with respect to hollow needle aspiration of cataracts, in the manner of the Arabic authors.[43] However, both Heister and Hirschberg seem to have missed the aspects of their descriptions related to pulling the cataract from the eye with a hook.

---

42 Feyens 1602, p. 30.
43 Hirschberg & Blodi 1984, vol. 3, p. 145–6.

Cataract Aspiration in Persia (1660)

Father Raphael du Mans (1613–1696) offered a satirical description of the oculists who aspirated cataracts in Isfahan, Persia, in 1660:

> Well then, concerning the physicians in Isfahan, I estimate that you will find more than fifteen hundred: *attars* or chemists, more than two hundred; *dellaks* (bloodletters, barbers), infinite quantity, one or two in each neighborhood; *gerrah*, there are a couple. Besides these, there are also oculists, *keihhal*, who do not allow old age to decrease vision: their trade is to treat the fools, who put themselves in their hands, by poking an eye or by blinding; for they do not know how to relieve the opaqueness of the eye. They blow multiple powders into the eye, like caustics that etch tunics and eventually make a stone and a wall of mortar. Upon this, to definitely prevent the optical ray to pass, they make use of a small syringe whose shaft is in a triangular shape: to the side and to the outer ends is a small aperture. They put it on both bruised [eyes] to evacuate the superfluous humour, that is what they say. They pull the small stick and by suction the ocular water enters this gutter. Hence the operation by our oculist. And they [*keihhal*] are even more ignorant than the three others [*attars, dellaks, gerrah*], who, since the diseases are usually chronic, suffice fairly for the country.[44]

This passage has been interpreted by some historians as representing removal of cataracts by aspiration,[45] which seems reasonable, given that the oculists of the Middle East believed the cataract to be caused by water in the eye. It is interesting that du Mans' writing confirms that of Shadhili that some oculists attempted to aspirate cataracts with suction produced mechanically, rather than with the mouth.

Cataract Aspiration in the Ottoman Empire (1655)

Evliya Çelebi (1611–1682) was a prolific traveler within the Ottoman Empire. His extensive writings have been only partially translated into English or German. Çelebi described eye surgery in southeastern Anatolia in 1655. To the best of our knowledge, this account has not been covered in the ophthalmology history literature.

Çelebi recorded that Abdal Khan, the Kurdish emir of Bitlis, in the present-day Turkey, performed cataract aspiration:

---

44 Du Mans 1890, p. 178.

45 Elgood 1970, p. 64.

> He is so skilled as an oculist [*kehhallik*] that he may take a man suffering forty years with cataracts [*gözine perde … inüp*, curtain] or glaucoma [*kara su inüp*, black water]: he inserts a bent hollow stylus through the inner corner of his eye, and when it reaches the back of the eye the Khan sucks the tube and brings out all the matter that has accumulated from steam, and the man's eyes become bright again, by God's command. Or to an eye with leucoma he applies Indian malachite and male collyrium and stork egg powder with a stylus, and removes the cataract like the peel of an onion. I have witnessed this myself.[46]

Khan was a true "Renaissance man": a ruler, a falconer, a tightrope walker, a musician, an architect, a bookbinder, and a painter.[47]

This account suggests that cataract aspiration did in fact continue in the Middle East throughout the medieval period, and into the early modern period.

Giuseppe Francisco Borri (1669)

Interestingly, it was during Çelebi's era that Western Europeans first claimed to be aspirating cataracts. Nearly 500 years passed between the first Latin and Hebrew translations regarding cataract aspiration before we find reports that Western Europeans attempted to actually perform the technique.[48] In addition, the first Europeans to attempt cataract aspiration did not cite these medieval Arabic authorities.

The first to claim that cataract aspiration was being attempted in Western Europe was Giuseppe Francisco Borri (1627-1695) of Italy, a religious heretic, alchemist, and sometime healer. By 1669, Borri had attributed the idea to an Italian surgeon named Rocco Mattioli, who served the archduke of Further Austria, Ferdinand Charles (1628–1662), whose court was in Innsbruck. A close examination of the potential for interaction of Borri, Mattioli, and the Ottoman Çelebi is quite interesting.

Borri began studying religion and medicine in Rome.[49] While there, in 1653, he also worked as a secretary serving Archduke Ferdinand Charles.[50] It may have been during his period in Rome that Borri became interested in the reconstitution of ocular humors after their experimental removal. In 1660, while in Rome, Giovannii Guglielmo Riva described removal of the ocular humors followed by their restitution with water of tetterwort (*Chelidonium majus*).[51] Borri later indicated (in 1669) that,

---

46 Çelebi, Dankoff 1990, pp. 96–7.

47 Çelebi, Dankoff 1990, pp. 96–7.

48 A somewhat ambiguous text from 1915 led to the myth that Ambroise Paré attempted cataract aspiration in the 1500s, but a close reading of Paré's texts shows that he did not mention cataract aspiration (Leffler "Çelebi" 2022).

49 Koch 2017.

50 Rotta 1971.

51 Koch 2017.

while in Rome, a nobleman from Naples communicated the idea of restitution of ocular humors with *Aqua Chelidoniae* to the Duke Orsini.[52] When Borri was declared a heretic, he sought protection from Archduke Ferdinand Charles in Innsbrook in 1658, where Borri remained until mid-1659, when he left for Strasbourg.[53]

By 1661, he had obtained a solid reputation in Strasbourg as a healer. He impressed the town with the cure of an ocular cancer in a painter named Otho, and he also filled the injured eye of a horse with fluids.[54]

By 1663, Borri had arrived in Amsterdam, where he demonstrated that after removal of the ocular humors in an animal, they could be replaced with his secret extract. That year, Danish scientist Ole Borch described the procedure ...:

> ... invented by Borri: He introduces a scalpel from above directly into the pupil of a goose, a dog, etc. Then, with his finger, he squeezes all the humours out of the eye, including the lens and the vitreous (as I have already seen twice with my own eyes). Then he pours a certain liquid, enriched with remedies, through a tube into the eye. ... Thus he fills up the eye to its previous round shape.... And, what a miracle - after nine days the animal is able to see again, and the humours that had been expressed are reformed.[55]

By 1669, Borri was in Denmark and continued to experimentally express the fluids of animal eyes by incising them and applying pressure to demonstrate restitution of the ocular humors.[56] However, in a 1669 letter, he also described a different type of eye surgery, namely, that Rocco Mattioli (or Roccho Mattioli) had performed cataract extraction by aspiration:

> I do not think I should omit here the mention of a rare instrument to remove cataracts of the eyes, invented by the noble lord Roccho Mattioli, Italian surgeon, formerly in the service of the Archduke Ferdinand Charles of Austria, whom I will never recall without tears to the pious memory of all the heroes and all the sages, as much because of his royal qualities as for the immense benefits of honors and riches with which he showered me. This man of art had imagined a needle in the shape of a reed, ending in a hollow point, with the aid of which he could penetrate into the eyes and extract the cataracts by applying suction to them with the mouth; but, as the narrowness of the orifice and the thickness of the membrane to be sucked embarrassed the ingenious artist in the operating maneuver, I myself advised him to enclose, in the brass tube of his needle, very fine threads of gold in the manner of a brush, which, being turned in a circle with the help of the fingers, while the needle occupied the center of the orbit, would emerge as from a sheath of brass,

---

52 Koch 2017.
53 Rotta 1971.
54 Koch 2017.
55 Koch 2017.
56 Koch 2017.

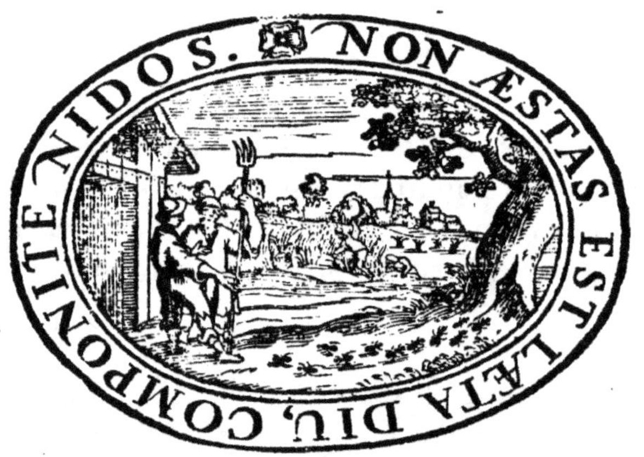

Fig. 5. Title page of 1671 appendix to Johannes Scultetus treatise, edited by Lamzweerde, which contains letter from Borri and figure of cataract extraction by aspiration (following page).

and would seize the membrane, or reduce it entirely to thin fragments, and, after having fulfilled this purpose, would be withdrawn within their brass envelope. The happiest result followed according to our wishes; in fact, the cataracts, displaced by this instrument, no longer returned to eclipse the light of the rays; while those which

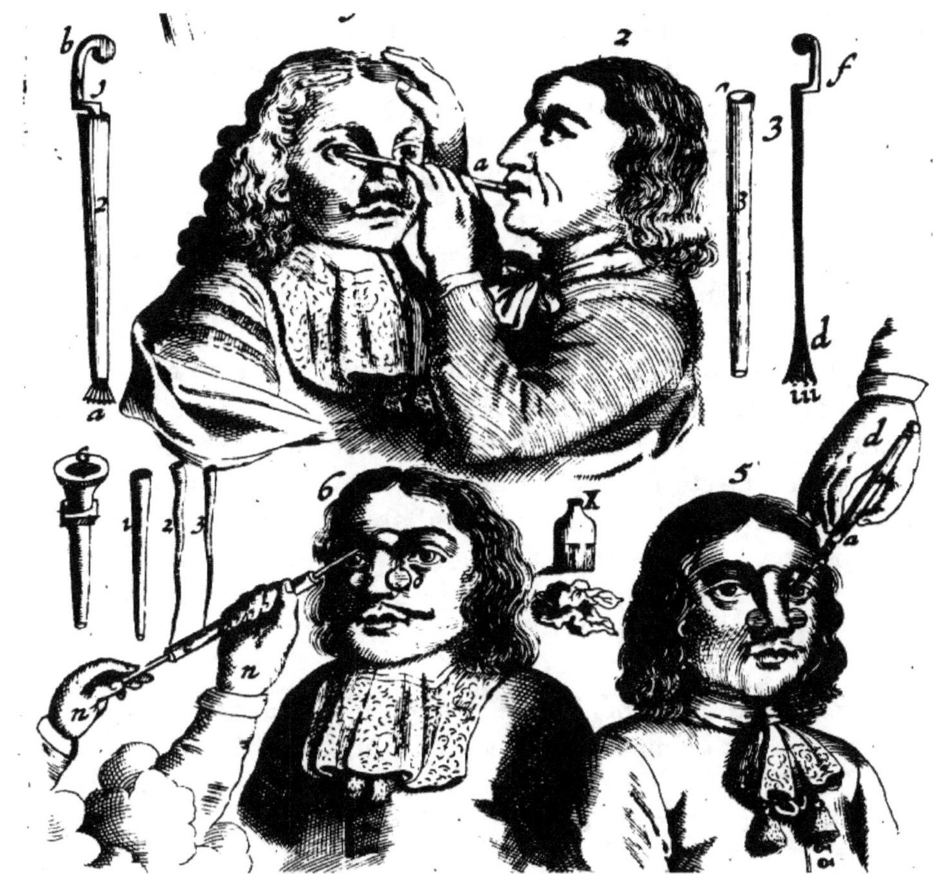

Fig. 6. Figure of cataract aspiration by suction, inspired by Borri's letter, drawn by the editor Lamzweerde of the surgical treatise of Johannes Scultetus.[58]

are lowered with the ordinary needle, are raised little by little by the movement of the eyes, as if they had not been completely torn from their roots.[57]

The illustration accompanying Borri's letter in the 1671 publication in Amsterdam focused on the part of the description related to aspiration (Figs. 5 and 6). However, if Borri intended that the brush inserted into the eye would pull on the crushed cataract debris in the manner of Scacchi's hook, then Borri's method was multifaceted.

Note the differences in surgical approach. Borri described a physiologic experiment in animals in 1663, but a treatment of pathology (presumably in humans) in 1669.

---

57 Malgaigne 1847, p. 191.

58 Scultetus, Lamzwwerde 1671, p. 62.

Borri described entry into the eye by incision in 1663 and by puncture with a hollow tube in 1669. Borri described removal of ocular contents by pressure in 1663 and by suction or grasping in 1669. He described removal of normal fluids in 1663, but removal of a pathologic membrane in 1669. (It should be noted that Borri, and most other Europeans, did not understand the cataract to be an opacified crystalline lens. Rather, they believed it to be a membrane anterior to the lens.) In short, Borri by 1669 is describing exactly the cataract aspiration technique that Çelebi attributes to the Kurdish leader Abdal Khan.

Also note that Borri does not credit the Greco-Romans or medieval Arabic authors with inventing the aspiration technique. Rather, Borri credits Rocco Mattioli who served the Austrian archduke. Could Mattioli have encountered Çelebi? As it happens, Çelebi was part of a diplomatic group who spent time in Vienna in 1665 working out a peace treaty between the Habsburg emperor Leopold I and the Ottomans. Çelebi spent a great deal of time at hospitals in Vienna. He described three surgeries in detail. Before a cranial trepanation to remove a wartime projectile lodged in the brain, Çelebi noted:

> The chief surgeon at the Stephen's cathedral hospital was to carry out this treatment. So I went straight to this master surgeon and engaged him in lively conversation.[59]

Amazingly, general anesthesia was used:

> The wounded man was given liquid resembling saffron to drink, and he passed out. Upon the man becoming intoxicated and unconscious, a fire was lit in a brazier and placed in a corner.[60]

The surgeon sat in front of the patient. Çelebi intuitively had a sense that the surgeon's breath could harm the patient:

> The surgeon asked why I was covering my nose and mouth with a handkerchief. "I might sneeze or cough, or just through my breathing a draft might enter the man's brain. I covered my nose and mouth to prevent that."
>
> "Bravo," he said. "A hundred blessings of God. If you were to study this science, you would become a master surgeon. And from the way you paid close attention when looking at the man's skull, I know that you have seen many things in this world."[61]

After the trepanation, the skin was closed with ants called "horsemen," which bit the opposing edges of skin together.[62]

---

59 Çelebi, Kreutel 1957, p. 127.
60 Bilsel 2012.
61 Çelebi, Dankoff, Kim 2010, p. 242–3.
62 Bilsel 2012.

Çelebi gave an overview of medical care in Vienna:

> There are a total of seven hospitals on the outskirts of Vienna for the sick. The largest and finest of all is the hospital at the Stephen's cathedral, in which all the couches and all the covers and sheets are made of brocade and silk and other fine fabrics, with costly gold embroidery. The Emperor [Leopold I] himself goes to this hospital, when he is sick.[63]

He also mentioned:

> There are such master surgeons in this city of Vienna, such excellent physicians and wise healers, <let every single one of them equal an E'û 'Alî Sînâ [Avicenna] and a Pythagoras ... Another day, when I visited <the hospital at the church of King László>, I made the acquaintance of an excellent surgeon from Cologne [KoLONYA], who could also speak a little Turkish. While I was writing down various words from the German and Italian languages, according to him, a jaundiced man who was bloated was brought in from the town of Istrenye in a cart.[64]

Did the city pronounced "KoLONYA" when rendered in Turkish correspond with Köln in Germany or the Cologne in Northern Italy, the home country of Mattioli?

Çelebi made specific note of the practice of ophthalmology in Vienna:

> But may the eternal Lord God protect this city from the rigors of war! Because if the enemy breaks into the city fighting, it will be destroyed. So may Allah allow her to surrender to Islam without a fight! Everything in this city is excellent and worthy of praise, but one must particularly praise all the healers and surgeons and blood-letters and ophthalmologists [*Augenärzte*], the painters and watchmakers and gunsmiths and turners ...[65]

In addition to the hospital at the cathedral, Çelebi observed a dental extraction performed: "One day, while I was sitting in a surgeon's shop ..."[66] Barbers worked in the surgeon's shops and shaved the head while sitting, unlike in Anatolia, where the barbers stood.[67]

---

63 Çelebi, Kreutel 1957, p. 126.

64 Çelebi, Kreutel 1957, p. 131, 245. Another translation of this section is: "while observing in a hospital in Monastir called King Lazlo, I became acquainted with a surgeon from Cologne who spoke Turkish fluently and could as well write other languages, including Italian and German." (Livingston 1970)

65 Çelebi, Kreutel 1957, p. 140.

66 Çelebi, Dankoff, Kim 2010, p. 244.

67 Livingston 1970.

Could Mattioli have corresponded with the doctors that Çelebi met in Vienna, or even met Çelebi himself? Presumably, Mattioli could have relocated after the death of his sponsor Archduke Ferdinand Charles in 1662. In fact, the Tyrolean line of the Habsburgs went extinct with the death of Sigismund Francis in 1665. That year, Innsbruck came under the direct rule of the emperor in Vienna, and the court of Ferdinand Charles, including musicians such as Antonio Pietro Cesti, relocated to Vienna. The daughter of Archduke Ferdinand Charles, Claudia Felicitas, married Emperor Leopold I in 1673. The widow of Ferdinand Charles, Anna de Medici, was present in Vienna by 1674. Both mother and daughter died in Vienna in 1676.

It is interesting to note that a century earlier, Pietro Andrea Mattioli (1501–1577) was a physician and botanist who died in Northern Italy (at Trento) and also served Habsburg royalty.

In 1670, Borri left Denmark, hoping to make his way to Istanbul in Turkey.[68] En route, he was captured and sent to Vienna, where he was imprisoned.[69] He detected an attempt to poison Emperor Leopold I with arsenic.[70] Borri was released by the emperor to face the charges of heresy by the pope only after guarantees were made that Borri would not face capital punishment in Rome, where he died of malaria in 1695.[71]

An illustration of cataract aspiration by suction accompanied Borri's description when published in Amsterdam by the editor Lamzweerde between 1671 and at least 1692.[72]

Dutch surgeon Anton Nuck (1650–1692) described paracentesis for hydrophthalmia in 1690. This technique of draining fluid from the eye by puncture with a needle was just entering Europe and had been inspired by Asian medical practices, including acupuncture.[73] In one case, after several attempts at standard paracentesis, Nuck reported:

> on the tenth day, having punctured the cornea (by inserting a thinner tube), we drew out as much aqueous and vitreous humour by sucking it out, so that it (the eye) differed little from its natural size ...[74]

This is the first therapeutic vitrectomy of which we are aware.

---

68 Koch 2017.

69 Koch 2017.

70 Koch 2017.

71 Marra 2022.

72 Scultetus, Lamzweerde 1671, p. 62; Koch 2017.

73 Leffler "hydrophthalmia" 2020.

74 Leffler "hydrophthalmia" 2020. Translations of the cases of Valentini, Nuck, and others who treated hydrophthalmia are contained in this chapter from 2020.

The diagram of suction of intraocular contents from the eye accompanying the surgical text of Scultetus continued to be published in Nuck's home country into the 1690s. However, the actual practice of suction of cataracts and vitreous apparently declined after this time.

Steven Blankaart (1685)

From antiquity onward, the cataract that was displaced by couching was believed to be an opacity, sometimes described as a membrane, which lay anterior to the lens. The lens itself was considered the seat of vision, as we might view the retina today. One of Nuck's colleagues was physician Steven Blankaart (1650–1704), who practiced in Middleburg and wrote a surgical treatise in 1680. According to the 1684 translation of his dictionary, Blankaart subscribed to the traditional view of a cataract as a pathologic membrane:

> the confirmed Cataract, is when the Pupil of the Eye is either wholly or in part covered and shut up with a little thin Skin; so that the Sun-beams have not due admittance to the Eye.[75]

The 1685 edition of Blankaart's surgical treatise proposed removing the cataract through a superior limbal incision:

> Chapter 8. About cataract … 16. After showing the current standards of treatment, I need to present my own thoughts as well. It is possible, I presume, to make a small incision in the upper part of the eye, above the *oogappel* [apple of the eye, complex of pupil and iris][76] and to extract the *valvlies* [membranous cataract] with use of two needles which are attached to each other like a pair of pliers: thereby there is no concern it [the cataract] will reappear. What is more, there is not so much trouble because of oozing of the fluids, since the laceration is above in the eye and it [the eye] is fixated. I reckon it is possible.[77]

It is interesting that Blankaart proposed a superior limbal incision almost a century before Benjamin Bell tested it in animals.

---

75 Blankaart 1684, p. 53.

76 Philippa 2003–2009; Schröder 1980.

77 Blankaart 1685, p. 64. Chapter 8, paragraph 16. Translation by Dr. Hogewind.

Gosky and Albinus (1695)

It is interesting that Feyens' work was published in Frankfurt, because the story continues in that city. In 1695, Leopoldus Dietericus Gosky defended a thesis depicting instruments for grasping a cataract and pulling it out of the eye through a hollow needle.[78] The preceptor was Bernhard Albinus, and Hirschberg believes Professor Albinus was the true author of Gosky's thesis.[79] Albinus was aware of Blankart's proposal but rejected it.[80] In any event, Gosky's thesis indicated that about 12 months earlier, an itinerant oculist who was undergoing an examination by the president boasted that he had a needle that could easily extract a cataract (Figs. 7–9). The needle had been sent to him by a friend from Riga, who had successfully used the needle. However, several months earlier, another oculist claimed to be the inventor of the needle and that the other oculist had mistreated him.[81]

Hirschberg explained that the thesis described "an elegant cataract needle, which, by pressing on a spring, could be opened like a forceps".[82]

Who were the two oculists in the story of Gosky and Albinus? We do not know. From 1692 to 1724, Johann Andreas Eisenbarth (1663-1727) from Oberviechtach practiced throughout Northern Germany.[83] However, he is not known to have arrived in Frankfurt until 1700.[84] His practice on the open stage was witnessed by the young Lorenz Heister.[85] Eisenbarth's troupe featured tightrope walkers.[86] A comedy played on his stage, but owing to its scandalous nature, the stage was destroyed by the authorities. Only one of the three blind patients Eisenbarth operated on could see to some extent afterward. In 1704, he claimed that two of the patients he operated on in Frankfurt could see afterward, and he advertised that one of his servants had escaped.[87] In 1705, he removed a bladder stone. He also performed surgery for hernias, cleft lip, and cancer.[88]

---

78 Gosky 1695, pp. 25–26.

79 Hirschberg & Blodi 1984, vol. 3, p. 146.

80 Hirschberg & Blodi 1984, vol. 3, p. 146.

81 Watson 1846, p. 59.

82 Hirschberg & Blodi 1984, vol. 3, p. 146–7.

83 Helm 1965, pp. 29–30.

84 Helm 1965, pp. 29–30.

85 Helm 1965, p. 30.

86 Henning 1989.

87 Helm 1965, pp. 30–1.

88 Henning 1989.

89 Heister, vol. 1, 1743, np.

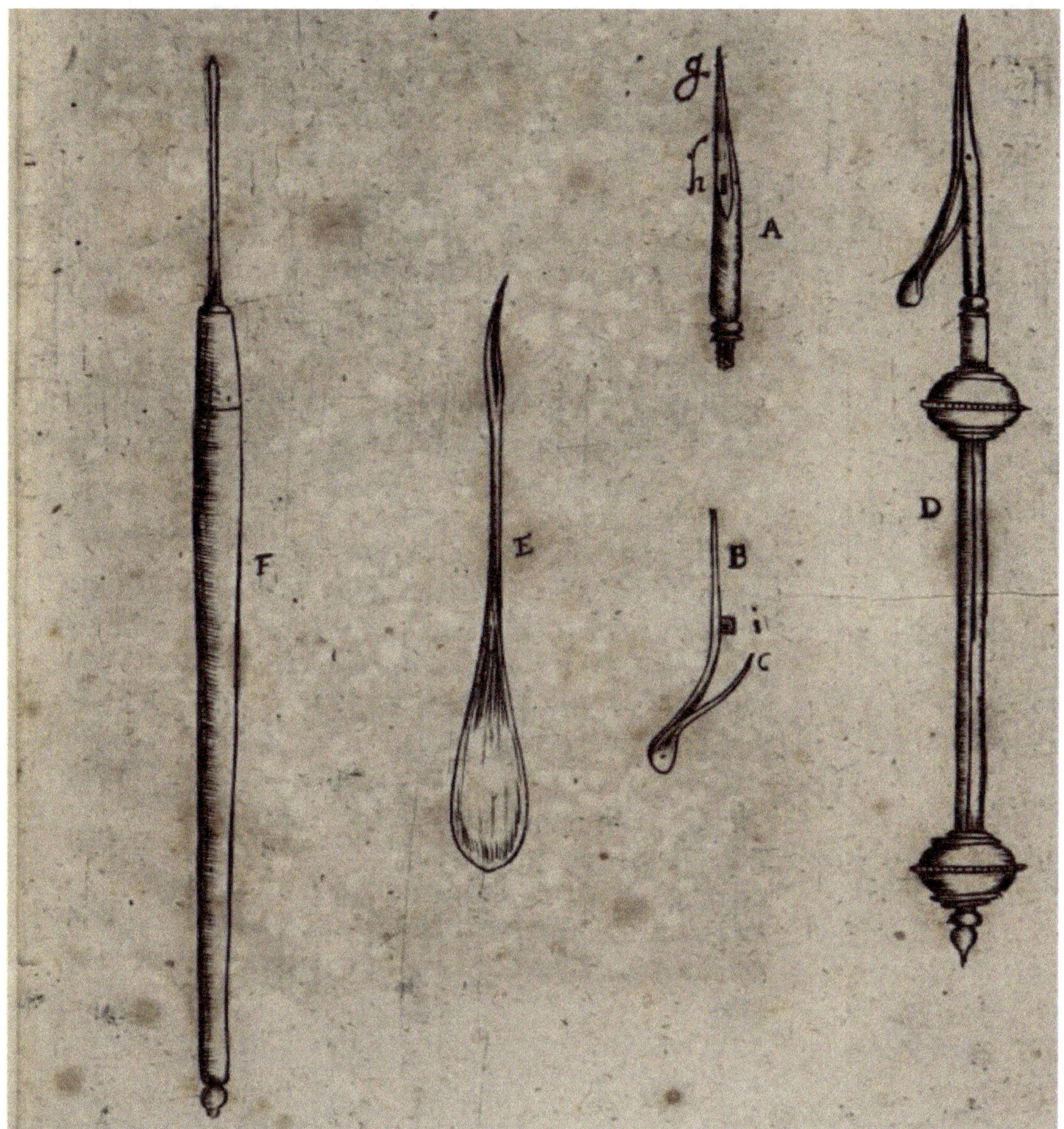

Fig. 7. Instruments for cataract extraction by grasping depicted by Leopold Gosky in 1695.

Thes. XV.

Annus circiter eft cum circumforaneus fe examinandum Domino Præfidi fifteret, qvi gloriabatur, fe acum habere quâ catarrhactam ex oculo commode educere poffet, eamqve fibi à veterano qvodam fuo amico Riga miffam effe qvi ea feliciter fuerit ufus. Sed ante paucos menfes alius qvidam agyrta fe primum inventorem effe profeffus prioremqve mala fide fecum agere teftatus fuit. Qvieqvid horum fit acum ipfam primo defcribam, qvidqve de ejus ufu fentiam fubnectam. D. Integram repræfentat, qvæ ex partibus A.B.C. componitur. A parsacus anterior eft, qvæ in cuspidem acutam, qvalem acus habere affolent, terminatur, non tamen uniformiter affurgit, fed in G incifuram habet ejus longitudinis & profunditatis ut B recipiat, ambæq; fimul acum efficiant rotundam: fumma induftria hæc poliri debent, ut animadverti non posfit è duabus partibus componi acum, ne fi alicubi promineat, dum in oculum intruditur, hæreat. H foramen eft in qvo I. obice firmatur, ut cardinem qvafi efficiant. C. elater eft, qvi utramqve partem tenet imobilem, ut non nifi digito preffæ recedant à fe & forcipem faciant, qvæ in manubrio D firmatur. Hoc modo præparata acu perforari oculum, cumqve ad

D   catarrha-

(26.)

catarrhactam pervenerit preffo digito elatere forcipe prehendi pelliculam, fimulqve extrahi debere volunt. Primo intuitu plaufibile eft rem ita confici poffe, acus enim ipfa tam affabre poliri poteft, ut cum qvalibet alia certet; qvicqvid tenacula prehenderis feqvatur oportet, ut pellicula è foramine facto commode extrahi poffe, aut fi in eo hæreat, firmari, ne redire poffit, debere videatur. Verum ut ut hæc largiar, nunqvam tamen in praxin vocari poterit: divaricari enim forcipis crura qvi poterunt qvæ in tunicis oculi hærent? qvæqvam folidæ & compactæ fint experientia docet, aut fi extrema vi preffo elatere crura deducere & foramen ampliare volueris, vel frangentur, vel exqvifitisfimos excitabis dolores, qvi ipfam operationem impedient & gravisfima deinceps fymptomata caufabuntur.

Thes. XVI.

Fig. 8. Gosky's description of cataract extraction by grasping the cataract.

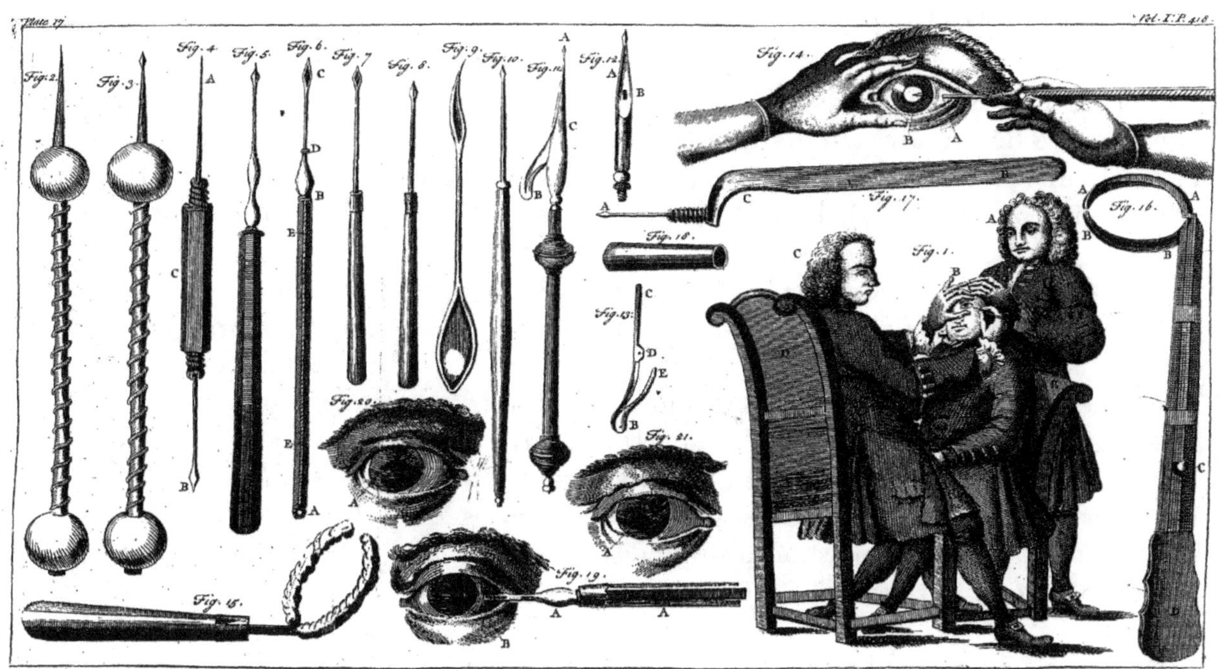

Fig. 9. Cataract instruments depicted by Lorenz Heister, including those from the thesis of Gosky under the supervision of Albinus (Heister's figs. 11-13). Heister summarized the use of Gosky's instruments: "*Fig. 11.* Denotes the Needle proposed by Albinus in his said Treatise, for extracting a membraneous Cataract out of the Eye; being so contrived that the Point A opens like a pair of Pliers in the Eye, by depressing the little Handle B; though I much doubt whether it was ever used with Success. *Fig. 12 and 13.* Represent the Parts of the preceding Needle separate and asunder. Fig. 12. Is the sulcated Point, in which is lodged the other Point Fig. 13. These perforate the Eye the better, as they are more exactly fitted and polished. They are connected by the Hinge B, C, D. Fig 11, 12, 13. E. Fig. 12. Denotes a spring to press the two points close together, till you open them by depressing it with your Thumb on the little Handle B Fig. 11. To apprehend and extract the Membrane."[89]

---

89 Heister, vol. 1, 1743, np.

Freytag (1698)

Johannes Conrad Freytag was a surgeon of Zurich who published in 1710 that between 1694 and 1698 he had drawn visual opacities out of the eye when an initial couching had failed, on at least three occasions. Johannes Conrad Freytag included these case reports in a book by Muralt in 1711.[90] In one case, Freytag reported (Fig. 10):

> The year 1694. It happened that the son of stable master Mr. Rinachers, who was learning the art of painting, by a strong emetic, which was given to him by a hangman, was affected so strongly, that he was blinded from that moment onwards and developed cataract ... It took half a year before they were ready [to operate]. I operated on both his eyes. Within eight days the cataract rose again, after which he only saw with the left eye. Again, I sent him away for half a year, in order to have the cataract curdled [clotted] and have it matured. Subsequently I operated the same again with a needle which had a fine hook (*häcklein hatte*) and drew the cataract out of the eye [*und zoge den Stahren aus dem Aug*].[91]

In one case, a 19-year-old who was born blind was cured by Freytag using couching in the usual manner. However, the patient then stole from Freytag's home, and an angry mob surrounded the patient/thief, grabbed his feet, and dragged him down the stairs, causing him to hit his head on the stairs. He was left blind again. After some time, Freytag used the hook-shaped needle (*häglichten Nadlen*) to restore the patient's vision yet again.[92] There is no indication from the account that the patient suffered from amblyopia, though that would be expected.

The third case with the hooked needle is interesting because it seems to have been used in a previously unoperated eye:

> In the year 1697, it happened that Mrs. RägeI Zuberin, age 40 years, in Eierbrecht near Zürich, developed cataracts in both eyes from a severe headache, when she was giving birth. I operated on one eye after several weeks in the old way with a smooth needle. Hereafter, she saw for an entire year, during which time, however, the cataract in the other eye progressed and grew. Then, the cataract in the seeing eye also rose again, upon which she did not see anything anymore. I operated on her again with a hooked needle in both eyes, attended by many local physicians, so she saw very happily and since then she is busy winding silk.[93]

Of course, Freytag does not specify explicitly in this passage that the hooked needle was used to draw the cataract from the eye, but perhaps he meant to imply that.

---

90 Muralt 1711.

91 Muralt 1711, pp. 29–30. This case was also discussed by Hirschberg & Blodi 1984, vol. 3, p. 35.

92 Muralt 1911, pp. 732–733.

93 Muralt 1911, p. 731.

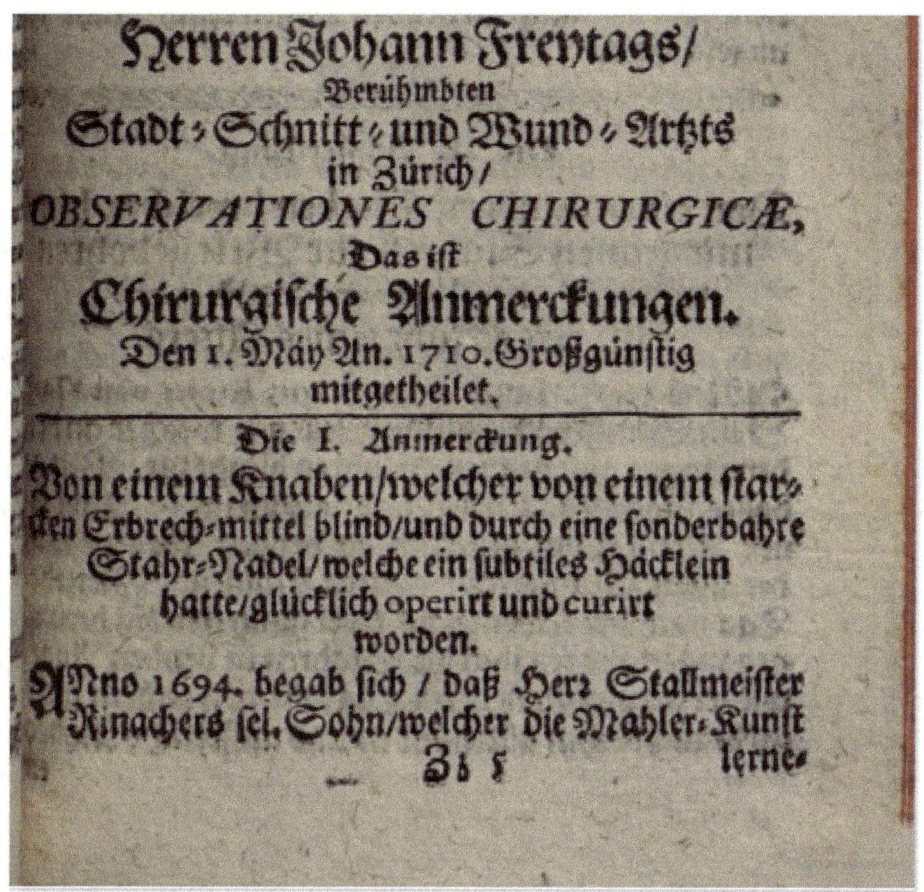

Herren Johann Freytags/
Berühmbten
Stadt-Schnitt- und Wund-Artzts
in Zürich/
OBSERVATIONES CHIRURGICÆ,
Das ist
Chirurgische Anmerckungen.
Den 1. May An. 1710. Großgünstig
mitgetheilet.

Die I. Anmerckung.

Von einem Knaben/welcher von einem starcken Erbrech-mittel blind/und durch eine sonderbahre
Stahr-Nadel/welche ein subtiles Häcklein
hatte/glücklich operirt und curirt
worden.

ANno 1694. begab sich / daß Herr Stallmeister
Rinachers sel. Sohn/welcher die Mahler-Kunst
lerne-
Z 5

730   Chirurgische

lernete / von einem starcken Vomitif, so ihm hiesiger
Scharfrichter gegeben/so starck beweget worden/daß
er von Stund an erblindet / und graue Stahren be-
kommen. Es verzoge sich ein halb Jahr/ehe sie zeitig
waren; als ich ihn an beyden Augen operirte/so stiege
der Stahren innerhalb acht Tagen an dem Aug wieder über sich/daß er nur an dem lincken Aug sahe. Ich
ließ ihn wieder ein halb Jahr gehen/ umb den Stahren wieder zu coaguliren/uñ erzeitigen lassen/operirte
denselben hernach wieder/mit einer Nadel welche ein
subtiles Häcklein hatte / und zoge den Stahren aus
dem Aug. Es wohnete sein Herr Götti/Herr Doctor
Lavate/ beyde mahl den Operationen bey / der Patient sahe demnach an beyden Augen etlich Jahr biß
an sein End.

Fig. 10. Johann Conrad Freytag's 1710 description of his 1694 cataract extraction using a hooked needle, published by Muralt in 1711.

In contrast, Freytag reported another cataract surgery, from 1695, using the conventional approach. In a 12-year-old boy who had been born blind, Freytag performed cataract couching "in the old way, with a smooth needle" (Muralt 1911, p. 730). After 2 weeks, the cataracts rose again, and his blindness returned. Fortunately, with medicines and time, the cataracts settled, and the eyes were clear and transparent.

In 1721, the surgeon's son, Johann Heinrich Freytag, also of Zurich, wrote a thesis on cataracts, which relayed his father's experiences performing cataract extraction by this technique. The younger Freytag claimed that his father had "performed several hundreds of cataract operations" but only a few with the hooked needle (Hirschberg & Blodi 1984, vol. 3, p. 35).

At the time, there was some controversy. Lorenz Heister asked his former student, Dr. Spoegel, to travel to Zurich to investigate. However, the younger Freytag refused to show him his thesis, or to perform the surgery despite being ordered by the directors of the hospital to do so (Hirschberg & Blodi 1984, vol. 3, p. 36). Muralt Jr. and Scheuzer said they had never seen a surgery like this. Spoegel declared the younger Freytag a liar. Hirschberg is perplexed that the investigator never examined Muralt's book, or spoke with the elder Freytag, who was still alive.

Subsequently, Heister also cast doubt on Freytag's work: "Mr. Freytage before-mentioned greatly recommends a Needle shaped like a Hook, for extracting membraneous Cataracts out of the Eye; but if this succeeds so well, why did he not give us the Figure of it?"[94] Later, Heister writes: "M. Freytage indeed advises to extract the Cataract, which he thinks is always a Pellicle [covering], by a Hook through the Cornea, as, he says, he has frequently seen done by his Father. But as he neither describes the Hook, or the Method of Extraction, and as I much doubt whether this Hook would not also extract or lacerate the Retina, Choroides and Sclerotica, 'tis, in my Opinion, best to neglect his Advice."[95] Heister also wrote:

> Those Surgeons who have persuaded themselves, that a Cataract proceeds from a Membrane or Tunic, have also provided themselves with an uniform Instrument, and extract the said Membrane through the Puncture made in the Coats of the Eye by the Needle, to prevent the Disorder from returning, as it might, if they were to leave the Cataract at the bottom of the Eye. Some of their Instruments were made tubular, in order to suck the Membrane from the Eye, others were made like a pair of small Pliers in the Shape of a Needle, as in Tab. XVII. Figure 10. and others again were like small Hooks which they introduced and extracted through a Cannula, together with the Tunic or Cataract, according to Freytage. But their Methods and Instruments were as useless and mischievous as their Notion of the Disorder was false.[96]

---

94 Heister 1743, vol. 1, part II, p. 410.

95 Heister 1743, vol. 1, part II, pp. 411–2.

96 Heister 1743, vol. 1, part II. pp. 414–5.

While the younger Freytag's response to the investigation seems a bit dodgy, he was judged too harshly by some of his contemporaries. The elder Freytag's description really did say that a hook-like needle was used for these opacities following cataract surgery, and in one case, the elder Freytag really did specify that the opacity was drawn out of the eye. If there was an exaggeration, the misstatement started with the father, not with the son.

Hirschberg debates whether the elder Freytag's cases related to an after-cataract or to the initial couched cataract rising again. Hirschberg thought these were entirely due to after-cataracts (secondary cataracts). However, in one case, the elder Freytag specified that he thought the cataract had risen again. Moreover, the case of the 19-year-old who became blind again after head trauma, but then could be restored with an eye surgery, also seems to relate to either the intact lens or residual lens cortex, moving into the visual axis. Head trauma could move opacities into the visual axis but could not cause a secondary cataract. Of course, secondary cataracts could have played a role in some of the cases.

Recognition of the Cataract as the Crystalline Lens (1705)

For many years, cataract surgeons would occasionally report that the lesion being couched was more substantial than a membrane. They may have adhered to the conventional (but erroneous) view that the cataract was an opacity anterior to the crystalline lens, but they knew the cataract was a round body with a surrounding capsule. For instance, Ammar of Cairo in the early 11th century observed that the cataract was a body with a capsule like that of an egg and that the capsule might be torn during couching without untoward consequences.[97] In 1622, Richard Bannister of England observed that couching could release a milky substance within the eye, which appeared to have been contained in the cataract, as in a "blather," that is, a bladder.[98]

Later in the 1600s, some French observers realized that a cataract was in fact an opacification of the lens. For instance, the idea was articulated by Antoine Le Grand (1629–1699) and contained in his translated and augmented treatise in English in 1694:

> Those that have a Cataract Co'ch'd, discern but obscurely all visible Objects; whereupon that they may the more clearly and distinctly see them, they make use of Convex Glasses. ... a Cataract is not any Skin (as hath been long believed) growing between the Chrystallin Humour and the Uveous Tunicle, which may be taken off by a Needle, and drawn down to the inferior part of the Eye, but that it is the Chrystallin Humour it self, which in tract of time grows flaccid and weak, and

---

97 Ammar, Meyerhof 1937, p. 41.
98 Banister 1971, pp. 54–7. Section "Of imperfect Cataracts".

> is separated from the Ciliary processes, as an Acorn when ripe, is easily separated from its Cup, forasmuch as it is removed with little or no trouble, and depressed to the very bottom of the Vitreous or Glassy Humour, a small part, in the mean time, of the said Vitreous Humour succeeding in its place.[99]

However, this idea did not initially achieve widespread circulation among surgeons.[100] It was perhaps inevitable that anatomic dissections would ultimately lead to an understanding that the cataract was an opacified crystalline lens. Alessandro Benedetti of Italy (c. 1450–1512) wrote: "How suffusions must be cured can be demonstrated in the eye of a cadaver."[101] Similarly, in 1521, anatomist Berengario da Carpi (1470–1530) encouraged the dissection of eyes with cataracts to further knowledge of this disorder.[102]

Several centuries later, a young French physician, Michel Brisseau (d. 1743), was skeptical of the ancient (but prevalent) teachings. Therefore, on April 7, 1705, he couched the cataract of a soldier who had died the previous day. Brisseau determined by dissection that the crystalline lens had been displaced into the vitreous. Brisseau's observation was read in the French Royal Academy of Science on November 18, 1705.[103]

By 1704, the French oculist Antoine Mâitre-Jan (1650–1730) had recorded several relevant observations, which were published in 1707.[104] When the cataract dislocated into the anterior chamber during couching, he noticed that it was thick and not a thin membrane. Mâitre-Jan noted the cataract to be an opaque crystalline lens at autopsy in patients who had been couched, and in others who had not.

Extractions of Anteriorly Dislocated Cataracts (1707)

Even before Jacques Daviel's work, some 18th-century surgeons would remove from the eye dislocated cataracts, which settled in the anterior chamber, often following a failed couching. On February 20, 1707, Charles de Saint-Yves extracted through a corneal incision fragments of a crystalline lens, which had spontaneously dislocated forward, producing inflammation.[105] This cataract extraction was performed in the presence of the French surgeon Jean Méry.[106] This procedure relieved the patient's pain.[107]

---

99 Le Grand 1694, p. 211.

100 Hirschberg & Blodi 1984, vol. 3, pp. 5–9.

101 Lind 1975, p. 123. Chapter XXXVII of *Anatomice of the History of the Human Body* (1502).

102 Lind 1975, p. 160. *Commentary on Mundinus*, 1521.

103 Hirschberg & Blodi 1984, vol. 3, pp. 10–15.

104 Hirschberg & Blodi 1984, vol. 3, pp. 18–19, 226.

105 Hirschberg & Blodi 1984, vol. 3, pp. 22,241; Duddell 1733, p. 30; Saint Yves 1741.

106 Méry 1888, p. 540.

107 Saint Yves 1741.

Another extraction of a lens that had dislocated into the anterior chamber was performed by the French surgeon Jean Louis Petit (1674–1750) on April 17, 1708, in the presence of Saint-Yves and Méry.[108] A "skillful English oculist,"[109] believed to be John Thomas Woolhouse,[110] was consulted. The Englishman proposed to meet the surgeons at the Academy of Sciences, to demonstrate that a membranous cataract had been extracted, but he failed to appear. However, on the appointed day, the patient and the extracted structure were examined, and the observers agreed that the patient could see with convex spectacles and that the crystalline lens had been extracted.[111] Woolhouse, in writing about the event, claimed that the patient was the one who failed to appear on the appointed day.[112] This case probably did the most to convince skeptics that the lens was not the seat of vision (as had long been proposed), because the patient was able to see afterward.

Saint-Yves described three cases of cataract extraction, including the two above, and a third in 1716. He performed this procedure whenever the lens became dislocated into the anterior chamber, and wrote: "I have formed many of these Operations."[113]

Woolhouse also accepted the extraction of intraocular opacities, although unfortunately for modern readers he used the term *cataract* for a membranous opacity, and the term *glaucoma* for an opaque crystalline lens. His precise description suggests that he may also have performed this procedure routinely when the lens happened to dislocate into the anterior chamber during couching:

> The tenth operation is when the cataract or glaucoma has passed into the pupil, between the cornea and the iris. It is called extraction of the cataract or glaucoma, and consists in a longitudinal section of the cornea, a little below the opening of the iris. The reason of making it here is, that as there will remain a dark cicatrix after the cure, the sight would be obstructed by it, more or less, if it traversed the front of the pupil.
>
> To perform this operation, the patient must be placed in the shade, where the pupil may be as much as possible distended: then planting the glaucomatic needle in the cornea, a line's distance from its outward circle on the temple side, and making it come out on the nasal side a line's breadth also from the circle; with a lancet made for the purpose, that must be no broader than a cataract needle, and cuts only on one side, make an incision according to the direction of the needle, the whole length of its entrance. The patient must be turned up on his back in the instant, without pillow or bolster, and the cataract or glaucoma drawn out of the first chamber of the eye, with an instrument made also for the purpose.[114]

---

108 Hirschberg & Blodi 1984, vol. 3, pp. 17, 266; Méry 1888, p. 540–1.

109 Méry 1888, p. 540–1.

110 Arrachart 1805, pp. 115–16.

111 Méry 1888, p. 540–1.

112 Saint Yves 1741.

113 Saint Yves 1741, pp. 261–66.

114 Woolhouse 1745, pp. 99–100.

English oculist John Taylor was rumored to have performed cataract extraction from the posterior chamber, according to Lorenz Heister, who wrote in 1739: "I have been assured from England, that this famous Oculist [Taylor] there boasted, that he could, and does extract Cataracts in this manner, which are even fixed behind the Pupil and Uvea; but I could never yet learn the Truth of his Assertion."[115] However, fellow English oculist Thomas Hope wrote:

> In regard to Taylor, he may have attempted, but never did carry it into practice; else he would not have fail'd to have publish'd it in the numberless productions he has given. I know, that, in 1743, I follow'd him in Edinburgh for six months, where he performed above 100 operations of the cataract by couching; but never once attempted this way, nor ever mention'd it, but in the case where the crystalline is lodged in the anterior chamber; which operation has been described by many authors.[116]

Duddell, Cleland, and Olivier (1733–)

In the 1730s and 1740s, several authors proposed cataract extraction by grasping or by suction, though they are not known to have followed through on these plans. In 1733, Benedict Duddell of England proposed a method to incise the cornea and extract cataracts by pulling them out with a hook.[117] However, there is no evidence that he actually performed the surgery.

Archibald Cleland (c. 1700–1771) of Bath, England published the design for several cataract surgery instruments in 1740.[118] The first was a cataract needle with attached forceps, used "either to depress a Cataract; or, if it should be found of such a Nature as to bear to be taken hold of, then, by opening the Points, to engage it, and carefully bring it out of the Eye."[119]

Cleland also designed a silver tube so that if couching was complicated by hemorrhage,

> it is so far introduced, as the End of the Tube is within the posterior Chamber of the aqueous Humour, the Needle is to be withdrawn, leaving the Tube in the Eye; and then, with the Mouth, may be sucked into the Tube, all the Blood, and watery Humour, that is contained there, or any other floating Particles. Then the Tube is to be withdrawn, and the Eye left to replenish itself with the aqueous Humour again; which will take Twelve or Eighteen Hours at most.[120]

---

115 Heister 1743, p. 416.

116 Hope 1752.

117 Duddell 1733, pp. 119–122.

118 Cleland 1740.

119 Cleland 1740.

120 Cleland 1740; Leffler "British Isles" 2021.

In 1751, Claude Joseph Olivier (1706–1780) presented in Lyons a new device he called a "Kenembatome," which permitted the surgeon "to apply the Syringe to the Tube, and suck out the Matter of the Cataract …"[121]

We have not come across proof that either Cleland or Olivier performed any cataract surgery, or that anyone actually constructed and used the instruments they designed.

Natale Giuseppe Pallucci and Jacques Daviel (1750)

An additional case of extraction of visual axis opacities from the posterior chamber was performed by Natale Giuseppe Pallucci in 1750. This case is particularly important in the history of ophthalmology, because it might have played a role in stimulating Jacques Daviel to forswear cataract couching and perform cataract extraction exclusively. The interplay of Pallucci and Daviel has not been previously written about. Daviel's publications and full-length biographies of Daviel do not even mention Pallucci.

Another surgeon who has been understood to have potentially influenced Daviel was John Taylor of England, who visited Daviel's hometown of Marseille in 1734. Daviel was living in Marseille in April 8, 1745, when he performed a difficult couching on Frere Félix, a hermit from Aiguille in Provence, near Aix.[122] This case demonstrated for him the limitations of cataract couching.

In fact, Daviel indicated a few years later (in September 1748) that the difficult couching in the hermit in 1745 motivated him to come up with a new manner of couching, which he conducted in seven patients between April 1745 and October 18, 1745:[123]

> I even dare to say that my new way of operating was so successful, that I immediately couched [*j'abattis*] seven cataracts with all possible success, & without any accident … You know the seventh patient whose cure done so much honor in Marseilles, where he came to me from Paris in the month of September 1745, to perform the cataract operation on him which he had had in his right eye for nine years … When he arrived in Marseilles, I explained to him the old method of operating on cataracts, and that of which I believe to be the inventor. I made him examine at the same time the instruments specific to the two methods, but above all, I did not let him fail to understand that I had only six examples to cite to him of those which were particular to me, and I asked him to be willing to decide in his own cause. He settled on my new method. So, I performed the operation on him on October 18, 1745.[124]

---

121 Leffler "British Isles" 2021; Garnier 1753, vol. 1, p. 115.

122 Daviel 1748; Daviel, Pearce 1967.

123 Daviel Sep 1748.

124 Daviel Sep 1748. "J'ose même advancer que ma nouvelle façon d'opérer fut si heureuse, que j'abattis sept cataractes tout de suite avec tout le succès possible, & sans aucun accident … Vous

Daviel's papers of 1748 and 1749 did not tell us exactly what this new couching technique involved. However, in 1752, he tells us what change he made in his couching technique in 1745:[125]

> I resolved to practice the traditional cataract operation with two instruments. The first was shaped like a small straight lancet, which served to open the sclera at the usual spot. The second instrument, shaped as a small spatula, was passed through this opening toward the top of the lens, to lie between this body and the posterior part of the iris.

This technique might have been new to Daviel in 1745, but it was not new to ophthalmology. Since antiquity, eye surgeons had dealt with the problem that the couching needle needed to be sharp enough to penetrate the sclera, but that a needle that was too sharp could damage the iris. Therefore, the ancients, such as Celsus, emphasized that the needle should be of intermediate sharpness. Beginning with the medieval period, Arabic authors, and perhaps unidentified Indian surgeons as well, used a two-instrument technique, as Daviel adopted in 1745, in which a sharp lancet was used to incise the sclera and then a blunter probe was used to couch the cataract.

Daviel moved from Marseille to Paris, arriving on November 7, 1746.[126] On June 24, 1747, Daviel received certificates from the military surgeons Sauveur Francois Morand (1697–1773) and Bouquot for cases of cataract couching, which Daviel performed in their presence at the Hôtel Royal des Invalides.[127]

Just a few weeks later, in July 1747, Natale Pallucci (1719–1797) was at the Hôtel Royal des Invalides watching Morand perform cataract surgery. Pallucci had been training in his birthplace of Florence in 1744[128] and later trained at Montpellier.[129] He moved from Montpellier to Paris in early July 1747.[130] Although Pallucci also wrote about lithotomy, he indicated that of all surgical disorders, those that

---

connoissez le septiéme malade don't la guérison m'a tant fait d'honneur à Marseille, où il me vint trouver de Paris dans le mois de September 1745, pour lui faire l'opération de la cataracte qu'il avoit à l'oeil droit depuis neuf ans … Lorsqu'il fut arrive à Marseille, je lui fis l'exposition de l'ancienne méthode d'operer la cataracte, & de celle don't je crois être inventeur. Je lui fis examiner en même tems les instrumens propres aux deux méthodes, mais sur-tout, je ne lui laissai pas ignorer que je n'avois encore que six exemples à lui citer de celles qui m'étoit particulieres, & je le priai de vouloir bien decider dans sa propre cause, il se fixa à ma nouvelle méthode. Je lui fis donc l'opération le 18 Octobre 1745."(Daviel Sep 1748)

125 Daviel 1967.

126 Daviel 1748.

127 Daviel 1748, pp. 21–22. Morand was Sauveur Francois Morand, Hirschberg & Blodi 1984, vol. 3, pp. 270–71.

128 Pallucci "Nouvelles remarques" 1750, p. 231.

129 Shastid 1918, vol. 12, p. 9215.

130 Pallucci indicated that he left Montpellier 2 weeks after a surgery performed on 23 Juin 1747: "Je Partis de Montpellier deu semaines apres l'Operation." (Pallucci "Nouvelles remarques" 1750, pp. 66, 68.

affect the eyes have always excited his attention.[131] He had tested in Italy cataract needles, which had a conical shape. However, within several weeks of arriving in Paris in July 1747, the military surgeon Morand had demonstrated for Pallucci a flat and sharp cataract needle that worked well.[132] Conceivably, Morand could have been influenced by watching Daviel perform cataract couching just weeks earlier. Pallucci devised novel instruments for lithotomy on cadavers with Morand at the Hôtel Royal des Invalides.[133] Upon his arrival in Paris, Pallucci must have heard from Morand about the cataract cures performed by Daviel.

Daviel attempted a couching in a wig-maker ("perruquier") M. Garion some time before Daviel's letter of September 30, 1748.[134] "Louis-Alexis Garion, *maître per-ruquier rue Dauphine*," had a 37-year-old son (born in 1711)[135] and, therefore, was probably an older person at the time of his cataract surgery. After the failed attempt at couching in M. Garion, Daviel incised the lower part of the cornea, held the incision open with forceps ("pincettes"), and introduced a needle ("aiguille") into the posterior chamber in order to draw the crystalline lens from the eye. This was accompanied by some loss of vitreous.[136] We do not know how large an incision was required to introduce the needle, or what cutting tools were used, because the description is brief. This case is considered the first ever documented extraction of a cataract from the posterior chamber (as opposed to the anterior chamber) in the history of ophthalmology. It was not a planned procedure, however. In his letter of September 30, 1748, Daviel wrote: "The observations which I made at this successful operation [on M. Garion] have aroused in me great ideas concerning the extraction of cataract."[137] Despite his obvious excitement, we will show that Daviel did not follow through on his interest in cataract extraction immediately after Garion's surgery.

Daviel later (in 1752) wrote that he had sometimes [*quelquefois*] practiced the operation of cataract extraction over the 3 years leading up to 1750 (*i.e.* from 1747 to 1750).[138] So, let us take a look at each of these periods.

First, we can ask about the later Montpellier and early Paris periods, that is, in Montpellier from November 1745, through his arrival in Paris on November 7, 1746, then until the end of June 1749. Did Daviel do any cataract extractions, other than for M. Garion, during this period? The answer is a resounding, "No!" Daviel never made that claim in his writings of 1748, 1749, 1752, or post-1752. Other than this extraction in the wig-maker Garion, all of the cataract surgeries performed by Daviel and detailed in his letters of September 1748 and of July 1749 were described as

---

131 Pallucci "Nouvelles remarques" 1750, p. X.

132 Pallucci "Nouvelles remarques" 1750, p. XI.

133 Pallucci "Nouvelles remarques" 1750, p. 81.

134 Daviel 1748, pp. 9–12.

135 Fehrenbach 2007, p. 42.

136 Daviel 1748, p. 11.

137 Shastid 1914, vol. 5, p. 3755.

138 Daviel, Pearce 1967; Daviel 1753.

cases of couching (*e.g.* "*...j'ai abbattu une cataracte...*").[139] He related the extraction in Garion as a singular event.[140] Daviel's presentation in November 1752 indicated that he practiced extraction *quelquefois* after Garion's failed couching / extraction but did not specify which months or years.[141] The undated manuscript covering cataract extractions from 1745 to 1752 confirms that Daviel performed no extractions between October 1745 and June 1749.[142] This manuscript also implicitly confirms that all of the cataract operations referred to in his letters of September 1748 and July 1749 relate to cataract couching, rather than extraction. On February 12, 1749, Daviel advertised in a Dutch newspaper that he resided in Paris and would take students interested in learning the technique he invented for reclination of cataracts using a new instrument (Fig. 11):

> hereby has advertised, that shortly he will start to offer private lessons on the ocular diseases, and that he will teach all the operations, which are needed for curing these, as well as a new operating procedure invented by him, in order to recline [*ligten*] the cataract, and the use of a new instrument to operate for it [the cataract]...[143]

The word used to describe the surgical action, *ligten*, was the archaic Dutch spelling for *lichten*, a term used to represent reclination of the cataract, that is couching in such a manner that the anterior surface of the lens faces superiorly as the lens lays in the vitreous.[144]

July 1749 marks a new period, because that is when Daviel published a letter responding to a critic of his couching technique.[145] And so, the next period we can analyze is from July 1749 through June 1750. Did Daviel perform any cataract extractions during this period? Perhaps. His undated manuscript claims that he performed cataract extraction from the posterior chamber in 15 patients between July 29, 1749, and the end of June 1750 (actually with the final surgery on April 17, 1750, in Douai).[146] Daviel's undated manuscript indicates that he extracted cataracts during this period in Paris, as well as in Auxerres, in the latter half of 1749; in Roye, Péronne, Cambrai, and Douai in April 1750.[147] There is some uncertainty, however, because he never published any names of patients or witnesses, or dates of surgeries, and never publicly claimed to have performed the surgery in any of these cities. Moreover, in the 250 years since, no doctors, patients, or family

---

139 Daviel 1748.

140 Daviel 1749, pp. 210, 221.

141 Daviel 1753.

142 André, Daviel 2005.

143 Daviel, 's Gravenhaegse courant, Feb. 12, 1749, p. 2. "*mitsgaders een nieuwe handelwyze by hem geinventeerd, tot het ligten van de Cataracta, en 't gebruyk van een nieuw Instrument om zulks te opereeren.*" "*Ligten*" is the archaic Dutch spelling for "*lichten.*"

144 Lindeboom 1985.

145 Daviel July 1749.

146 Andre, Daviel 2005.

147 André, Daviel 2005.

De Heer DAVIEL, wonende op de Malaquay-Kade te Parys, digt by 't Hôtel van Bouillon, in 't Huys van den Heer Requeſtmeeſter Mondot, bevorens geweezen Chirurgyn van de Galeyen te Marſeille, dog nu zeedert den eerſten January van dit jaer 1749 door den Koning van Vrankryk benoemd tot zynen CHIRURGYN-OCULIST, welke Charge een geruymen tyd vacant was geweeſt, vermits het overlyden van den Heer *Pierre Parthon*, den laetſten Bezitter, zynde hy Heer DAVIEL ordinaris Chirurgyn van den Koning *par quartier by Survivance*; dezelve, die geſchreeven heeft de Miſſive, geinſereerd in de Mercurius van de maend September 1748, pag. 198, aen den Heer *de Joyeuſe*, Doktor van 's Konings Hofpitalen te Marſeille geadroſſeerd; wiens Antwoord daer op is te vinden in 't Iſte Vol. van de Mercurius van de maend December daer aen volgende, pag. 168, doet by deezen adverteeren, dat hy binnen korten zal beginnen particuliere Leſſen te geeven over de *Oogen-quaelen*, en dat hy zal onderwyzen alle de operatien, tot geneeſinge derzelver vereyſcht werdende, mitsgaders een nieuwe handelwyze by hem geinventeerd, tot het ligten van de *Cataratta*, en 't gebruyk van een nieuw *Inſtrument* om zulks te opereeren. De gem. Heer DAVIEL heeft goed Logement voor de perſonen, die door hem van hunne Oog-quaelen verlangen geneeſen te zyn, en neemd Leerlingen, om die te onderwyzen, in de koſt.

GERRIT TEN NAERDEN, maekt en verkoopt alle zoorten van Kamer…

Fig. 11. Daviel's advertisement in the *Gravenhaegse courant*, February 12, 1749, announcing that he reclines (*ligten*) the cataract.

… cette Académie doit ſon Etabliſſement.

FRANCE.

De PARIS *le* 16. *Mars.*

M. le Marechal Duc de Richelieu, qui eſt … en *Languedoc*, ſera, dit-on, nommé pour accompagner S. A. R. l'Infante Dona … Antoinette, future Epouſe du Duc de …, lorſque cette Princeſſe traverſera la … pour ſe rendre à *Turin*; & l'on aſſure … ce Seigneur ſe rendra enſuite à *Genes*. … paroît un Arrêt du Conſeil d'Etat du Roi … à 6. mois pour tout delai, le Viſa des … concernant l'ancienne Compagnie de la

* On donne avis que Mr. Daviel, Conſeiller ordinaire & Oculiſte du Roi Très Chretien, partira de cette Ville le 18. de ce mois pour ſe rendre à *Petersbourg*. S. M. permet à ce Chirurgien de voyager pour le bien du Public: Il paſſera par *Senlis, Peronne, Cambrai, Arras, Doüay, Bethune, Lille, Dunkerque* & par toutes les principales Villes de *Flandres* & de *Brabant*, & ſejournera dans chacune d'icelles: Il ira enſuite à *Londres*; de là il paſſera en *Hollande*, puis en *Allemagne*, en *Pruſſe*, en *Saxe*, en *Pologne* & enfin en *Ruſſie*: Mr. Daviel a fait pluſieurs Decouvertes heureuſes ſur les Maladies des Yeux & un très grand nombre d'Operations très difficiles qui lui ont parfaitement réüſſi: Il ſe flatte qu'il ne dementira pas dans le Païs étangers la Reputation qu'il s'eſt acquiſe dans le ſien.

Fig. 12. Daviel's March 16 announcement in the *Gazette d'Amsterdam* of March 24, 1750, that he will leave Paris on March 18 and travel to London and St. Petersburg.

members have come forward to support Daviel's unpublished claims. Perhaps, more could be learned from biographical research of the names in Daviel's unpublished manuscript, as well as in newspaper accounts.

If Daviel did perform cataract extractions without telling anyone during this period, then it was a time when he was still honing his craft. His unpublished log lists most cases as successful (*bien réussi*), but he has several failures during this early period. For two successive surgeries in Paris, both of which were bilateral, and the first of which took place on February 4, 1750, the outcome was listed as *dans un n'a pas réussi*. Likewise, the surgery in Douai on April 17, 1750, was listed as *mal réussi*.[148]

As can be noted from Daviel's itinerary, he left Paris in the spring of 1750. In fact, he planned to take a grand sojourn, to the Low Countries, to England, to Germany, Vienna, Poland, and St. Petersburg. He announced his tour from Paris on March 16, 1750 (Fig. 12):

---

148 Andre, Daviel 2004.

> Notice is given that Mr. Daviel, *Conseiller ordinaire & Oculiste du Roi Très Chretien*, will leave this City on the 18th of this month to go to St. Petersburg. His Majesty allows this Surgeon to travel for the good of the Public: He will pass through Senlis, Perronne, Cambrai, Arras, Douay, Bethune, Lille, Dunkirk & through all the main Cities of Flanders & Brabant, & will stay in each of them: He will then go to London; from there he will go to Holland, then to Germany, to Prussia, to Saxony, to Poland & finally to Russia: Mr. Daviel has made several happy Discoveries on Eye Diseases & a very large number of very difficult Operations which have perfectly successful: He flatters himself that he will not deny in foreign countries the reputation he has acquired in his own.[149]

There is no hint in Daviel's notice that he has discovered a single revolutionary innovation in cataract surgery and that he intends to remain in France to have a new surgical technique evaluated by his peers and the Academy of Surgery.

By March 23, 1750, Daviel had decided to delay his trip for a few weeks.[150] On April 21, 1750, it was announced from Paris that Daviel had not been able to leave the city until April 5 because he had multiple operations to perform there and that he was now delayed en route due to his high volume of operations.[151] Thus, it seems Daviel had some communication with contacts in Paris during his journey.

Daviel visited Cambrai in the spring of 1750, and in his unpublished manuscript, he later claimed to have performed cataract extractions in two patients successfully on that visit. The magistrate of Cambrai wrote a letter to the secretary of state of that town on May 9, 1750, lauding "le sieur Daniel [sic], chirurgien et oculiste ordinaire du roy" for succeeding in the vast majority of his operations for cataract, inflammation, and other eye conditions.[152] There is nothing in the magistrate's letter or the secretary's response to suggest that two of Daviel's cataract operations used a newer technique.

The autumn of 1750 was to be transformative for ophthalmology. So, what happened just before that period? When Europe's most famous composer, Johann Sebastian Bach, died in Leipzig on July 28, 1750, at least some newspapers blamed the English

---

149 Daviel, Gazette d'Amsterdam: March 24, 1750. "Paris, le 16 Mars. On donne avis que Mr. Daviel, Conseiller ordinaire & Oculiste du Roi Très Chretien, partira de cette Ville le 18. De ce mois pour se rendre à Petersbourg. S. M. Permet à ce Chirurgien de voyager pour le bien du Public: Il passera par Senlis, Perronne, Cambrai, Arras, Douay, Bethune, Lille, Dunkerque & par toutes les principals Villes de Flandres & de Brabant, & sejournera dans chacune d'icelles: Il ira ensuite à Londres; de là il passera en Hollande, puis en Allegmagne, en Prusse, en Saxe, en Pologne & enfin en Russie: Mr. Daviel a fait plusieurs Decouvertes heureuses sur les Maladies des Yeux & un très grand nombre d'Operations très difficiles qui lui ont parfaitement réussi: Il se flatte qu'il ne dementira pas dans le Païs étangers la Reputation qu'il s'est acquise dans le sien."

150 Daviel, Gazette d'Amsterdam: March 31, 1750.

151 Daviel, Gazette d'Amsterdam: April 28, 1750.

152 Coulon 1908, p. 176.

oculist John Taylor, who had performed an eye surgery on Bach in the spring of that year. The *Spenersche Zeitung* called Bach's death "an unfortunate consequence of an operation very badly performed on his eyes by a well-known English oculist."[153] This was not a point in favor of traditional cataract couching, though it is doubtful that Taylor really caused Bach's death, and there is no evidence that Daviel was impacted by this news story.

In 1750, Pallucci devised several innovations in cataract surgery while in Paris. As noted earlier, many surgeons since the medieval period, including Daviel, performed couching with a two-instrument technique: a sharp lancet to incise the sclera and then a blunter probe to couch the lens without damaging the iris. Pallucci's needle, in a work he signed April 27, 1750 (and published May 12, 1750), avoided the need to use two separate instruments (Fig. 13). It involved a combination needle within a tubule. When the needle was in place, the device was used to perforate the sclera. Then, the needle was withdrawn into the tubule, leaving in the scleral perforation the blunt tubule with which the operation was completed.[154]

Pallucci also published an account of six former soldiers operated for cataract at the Hôtel Royal des Invalides in the spring of 1750, with the cases assisted by the military surgeon Morand, often with Bouquot witnessing as well.[155] On May 11, 1750, Pallucci performed a cataract couching on an older soldier named Charles Pagliano in Paris.[156] However, an opacity that Pallucci believed to be the lens capsule returned to the visual axis and was located behind the pupil (*place derriere la prunelle ... etoit la Capsule du Crystallin*).[157] Pallucci on July 3, 1750, used forceps (*pincettes*) to extract the detached capsule and fragments of the cataract (*plusiers fragmens*) from the posterior chamber after making a corneal incision (Fig. 14).[158] Morand certified on August 25, 1750, that Pallucci had "new ideas" (*des idées neuves*) on the cataract operation.[159] Pallucci recorded these cases on August 29, 1750, and his book was registered on September 5, 1750.[160]

Right after Pallucci's July 3, 1750, after-cataract extraction, we see a number of changes in Daviel's surgical practice. The first change is that Daviel begins performing experiments related to cataract extraction on animals. In his entire unpublished log of human and animal cataract extractions, running for 8 years, from April 1745 to the end of 1752, Daviel only performed animal work for 4 months: from July to November 1750. Daviel's first animal experiment was on a sheep on July 7,

---

153 Lenth 1938.

154 Pallucci "Nouvel Instrument" 1750; Shastid 1918, vol. 12, p. 9215; Hirschberg & Blodi 1984, vol. 3, p. 393.

155 Pallucci "Histoire" 1750, pp. 10,19,53,56.

156 Pallucci "Lettre" 1751, p. 31.

157 Pallucci "Histoire" 1750, p. 37.

158 Pallucci "Histoire de l'operation" 1750, p. 39.

159 Pallucci "Histoire" 1750, pp. 55–56.

160 Pallucci "Histoirc" 1750, pp. 43, 56.

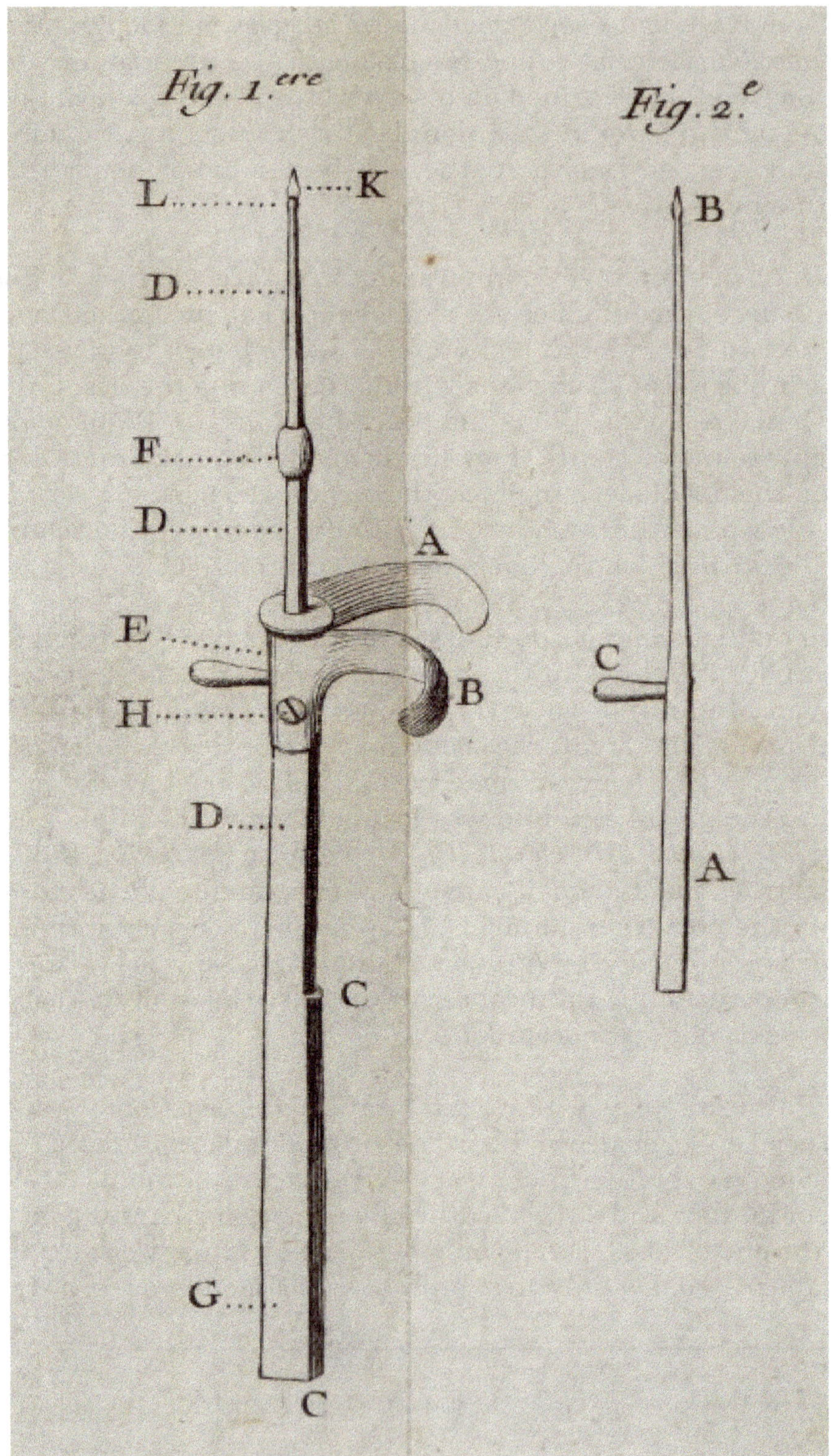

Fig. 13. A combination needle–cannula for cataract surgery that Pallucci published in a work he signed April 27, 1750.

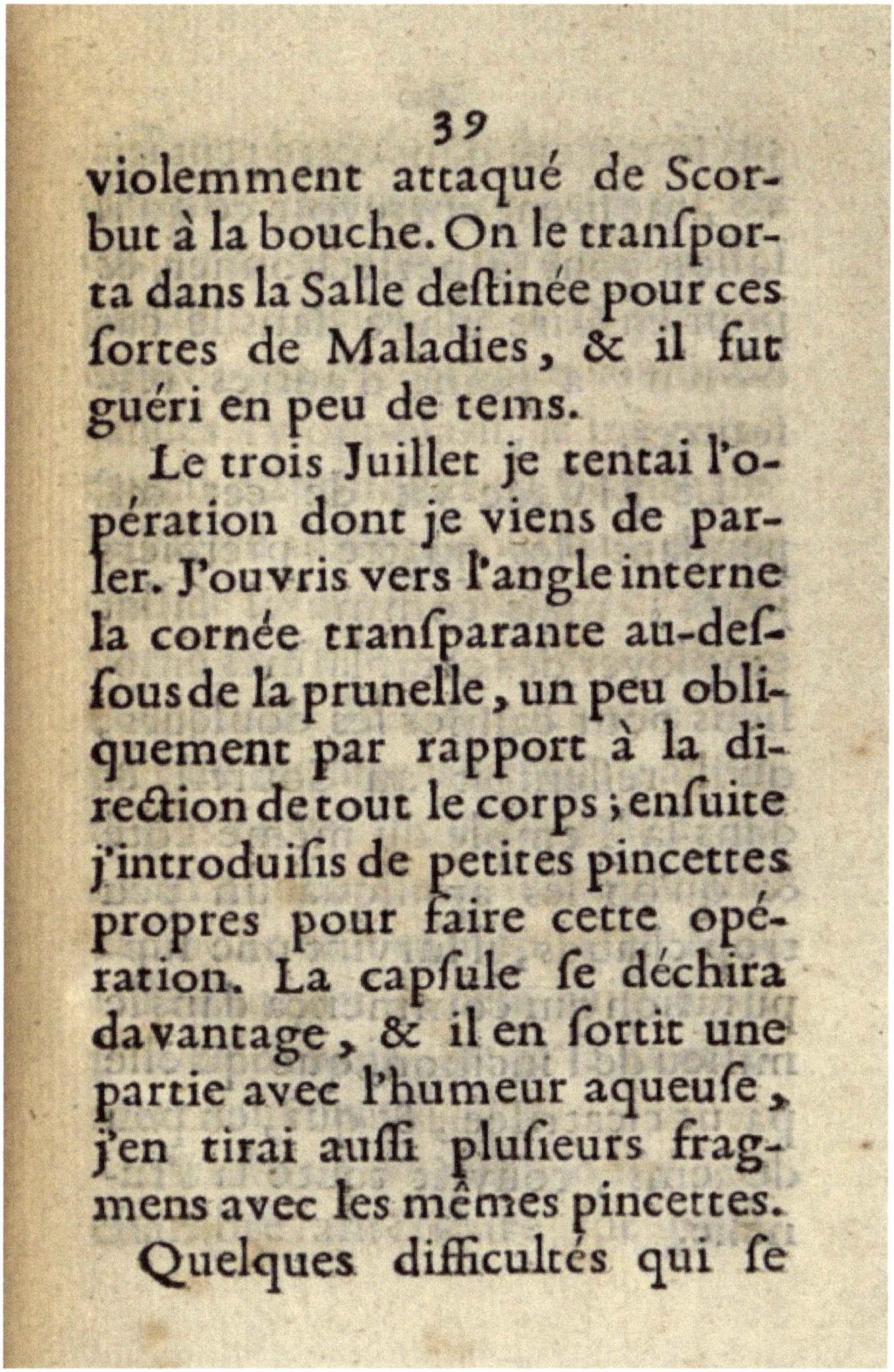

39

violemment attaqué de Scor-
but à la bouche. On le tranſpor-
ta dans la Salle deſtinée pour ces
ſortes de Maladies, & il fut
guéri en peu de tems.

Le trois Juillet je tentai l'o-
pération dont je viens de parler. J'ouvris vers l'angle interne
la cornée tranſparante au-deſ-
ſous de la prunelle, un peu obli-
quement par rapport à la direction de tout le corps; enſuite
j'introduiſis de petites pincettes
propres pour faire cette opération. La capſule ſe déchira
davantage, & il en ſortit une
partie avec l'humeur aqueuſe,
j'en tirai auſſi pluſieurs fragmens avec les mêmes pincettes.
Quelques difficultés qui ſe

Fig. 14. Pallucci on July 3, 1750, used forceps (*pincettes*) to extract the detached capsule and fragments of the cataract from the posterior chamber after making a corneal incision.

1750: *A Louvin Deux expériences faites sur des yeux de Mouton le 7 Juillet.*[161] This experiment was conducted in between Daviel's stops in Douai and Liège. And so, Daviel conducted his first animal experiments on cataract extraction 4 days after Pallucci's surgery, and about 200 miles away. Perhaps, Daviel's animal work was begun in response to Pallucci's surgery, or perhaps it was begun because the immediately previous surgery in Douai in April 1750 had failed. Daviel continued to perform animal experiments on cataract extraction on a dog in Liège on August 12, 1750; on a sheep in Cologne in September 1750 in the presence of the faculty; on a sheep on November 3, 1750, in Mannheim; and then on the horse of the Elector on November 12, 1750, in front of a prince.[162] This period of animal experimentation, which is not found over any other time in the record from 1745 to 1752, supports the idea that the period from July to November 1750 was one of innovation for Daviel.

Another change in Daviel's practice in the latter half of 1750 is that he is willing to go on record stating the cities in which he performed the cataract extractions. As we will see, Daviel later published some vague claims about performing cataract extractions many years previously, but he did not say in what city he performed the surgeries, or in what year. So, the claims were completely unfalsifiable. Daviel's peers could not go to any particular city and ask the doctors there if they had heard about the cases. But with respect to the extractions Daviel performed in the latter half of 1750, he named the cities in his 1752 presentation to the Academy of Surgery: Liège, Cologne, and Mannheim. In 1752, any of Daviel's peers could have gone to the doctors in these cities to verify what happened 2 years earlier.

However, there is an even stronger reason to believe that Daviel really performed planned cataract extraction from the posterior chamber in the fall of 1750: It was documented contemporaneously in the newspapers and by other witnesses. These newspaper accounts have seemingly not been noticed by historians.

Daviel later wrote that in Liège, he performed six cataract extractions in four patients, between July 22 and August 17, 1750.[163] That might be possible, but we have not found newspaper notices to confirm this. In fact, the initial newspaper accounts just seem to say that he is a good ophthalmologist, without hinting at any revolutionary changes.

On July 26, 1750, the Regensburg newspaper reported that Germany was full of oculists: "Taylor, Cyrus, Illert, Hillmer, Mainerts." Likewise, "Oculisten, Herrn Daviel" arrived in Liège on July 18, 1750, and has permission to practice his art. He intends to travel to "Cölln, Frankfurt, Nurnberg, Regenspurg" and then on to Vienna (Fig. 15).[164]

---

161 Andre, Daviel 2005; The handwriting could be "Aversin" (Haversin), which is also between Douai and Liege, and is also 200 miles from Paris.

162 Andre, Daviel 2005.

163 Daviel, Pearce 1967; Andre, Daviel 2005.

164 [No author listed], Staats-Relation, vol. 6, 1750, p. 355.

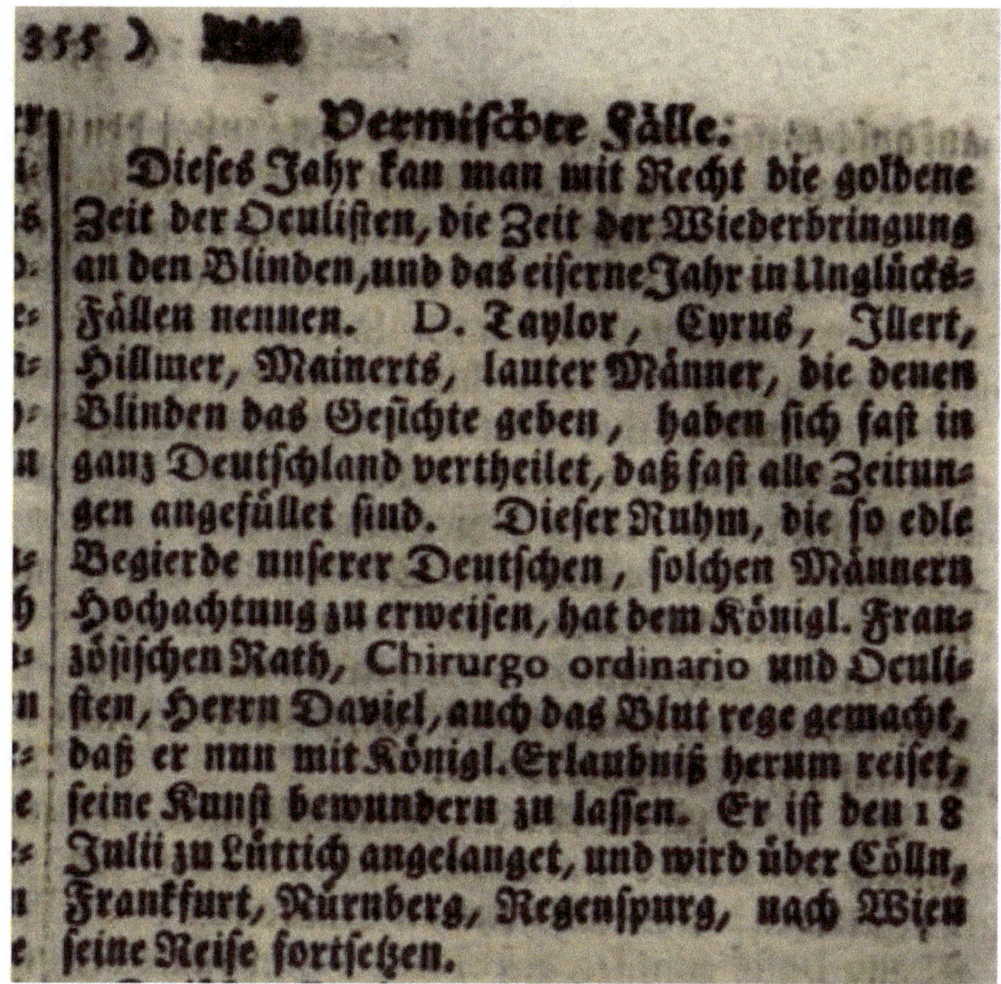

Fig. 15. The Regensburg newspaper *Staats-Relation der neuesten europäischen Nachrichten und Begebenheiten* of July 26, 1750, announced that Daviel was practicing in Liège.

On August 30, 1750, the Regensburg newspaper noted that the "Chirurgien Ordinaire und Oculiste Daviel" is in Liège and distinguishes himself from many others by his operations on the eyes and in other types of surgical operations. He operates on the poor free of charge and stays in one place until the patients have recovered (see Figure 16).[165] These seem to be just good ophthalmology practice, rather than revolutionary innovations (Fig. 16).

On September 16, 1750, the Regensburg newspaper noted that Daviel had arrived in Cologne and would arrive in Vienna soon (Fig. 17).[166]

---

165 [No author listed], Staats-Relation, vol. 6, 1750, p. 415.
166 [No author listed], Staats-Relation, vol. 6, 1750, p. 444.

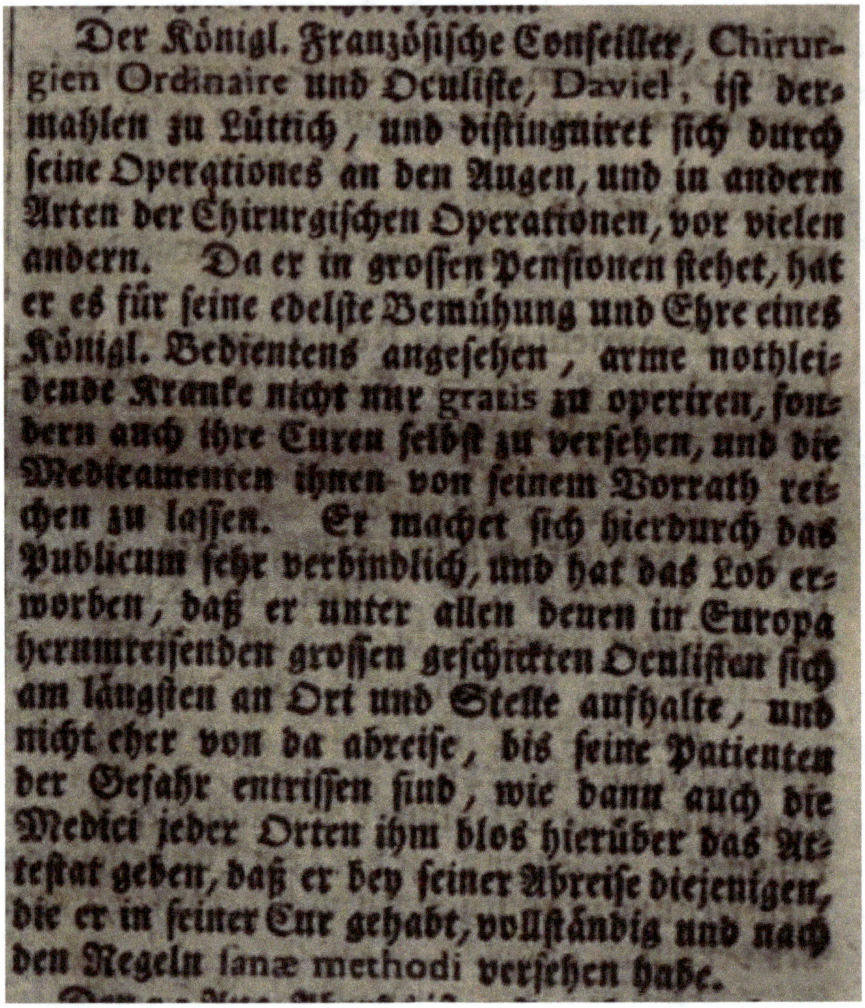

Der Königl. Französische Conseiller, Chirurgien Ordinaire und Oculiste, Daviel, ist der-
mahlen zu Lüttich, und distinguiret sich durch
seine Operationes an den Augen, und in andern
Arten der Chirurgischen Operationen, vor vielen
andern. Da er in grossen Pensionen stehet, hat
er es für seine edelste Bemühung und Ehre eines
Königl. Bedientens angesehen, arme nothlei-
dende Kranke nicht nur gratis zu operiren, sondern auch ihre Curen selbst zu versehen, und die
Medicamenten ihnen von seinem Vorrath rei-
chen zu lassen. Er machet sich hierdurch das
Publicum sehr verbindlich, und hat das Lob erworben, daß er unter allen denen in Europa
herumreisenden grossen geschickten Oculisten sich
am längsten an Ort und Stelle aufhalte, und
nicht eher von da abreise, bis seine Patienten
der Gefahr entrissen sind, wie dann auch die
Medici jeder Orten ihm blos hierüber das At-
testat geben, daß er bey seiner Abreise diejenigen,
die er in seiner Cur gehabt, vollständig und nach
den Regeln sanæ methodi versehen habe.

Fig. 16. The Regensburg newspaper *Staats-Relation der neuesten europäischen Nachrichten und Begebenheiten* of August 30, 1750, announced that Daviel still practiced in Liège.

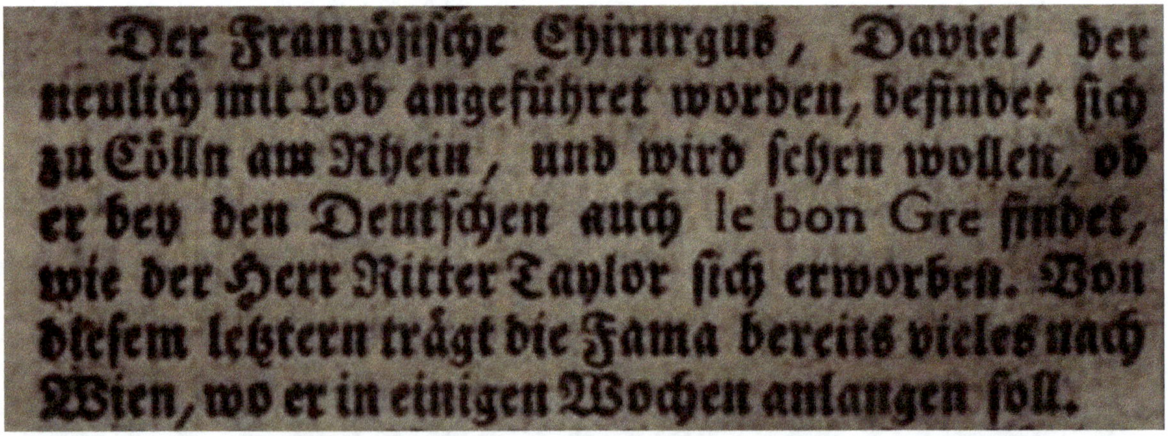

Der Französische Chirurgus, Daviel, der
neulich mit Lob angeführet worden, befindet sich
zu Cölln am Rhein, und wird sehen wollen, ob
er bey den Deutschen auch le bon Gre findet,
wie der Herr Ritter Taylor sich erworben. Von
diesem letztern trägt die Fama bereits vieles nach
Wien, wo er in einigen Wochen anlangen soll.

Fig. 17. The Regensburg newspaper *Staats-Relation der neuesten europäischen Nachrichten und Begebenheiten* of September 16, 1750, announced that Daviel had arrived in Cologne.

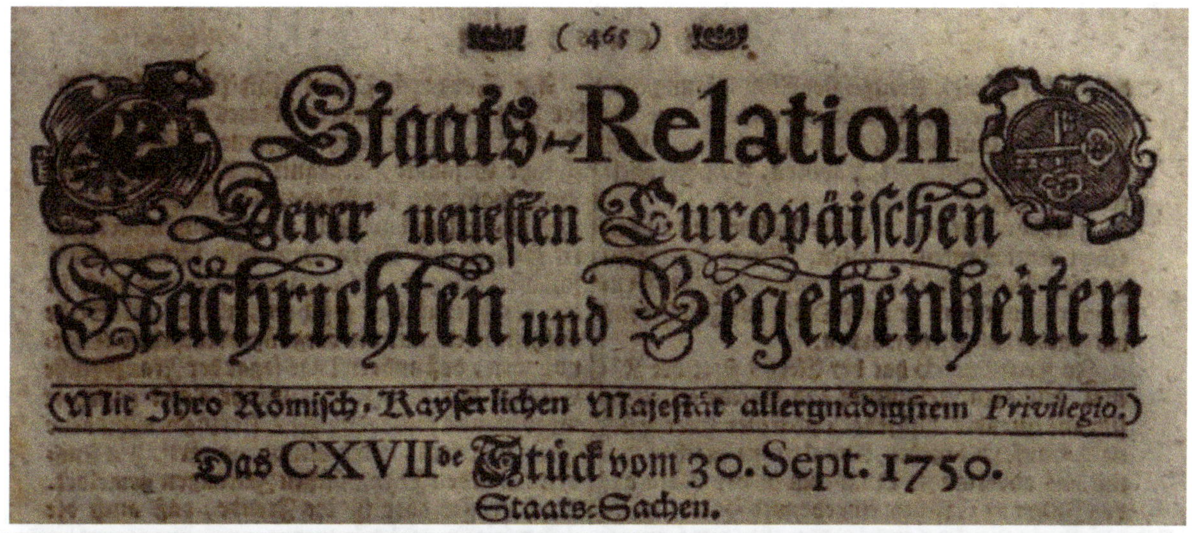

Fig. 18. A and B. The Regensburg newspaper *Staats-Relation der neuesten europäischen Nachrichten und Begebenheiten* of September 30, 1750, announced that Daviel has performed a cataract extraction on Franciscan father Nouprez in Cologne.

According to Daviel's log, he only performed one cataract extraction in Cologne,[167] and we see the revolutionary nature of this particular case hailed in the Regensburg newspaper of September 30, 1750:[168]

---

167 Andre, Daviel 2004.

168 [No author listed] Staats-Relation, vol. 6, 1750, p. 468.

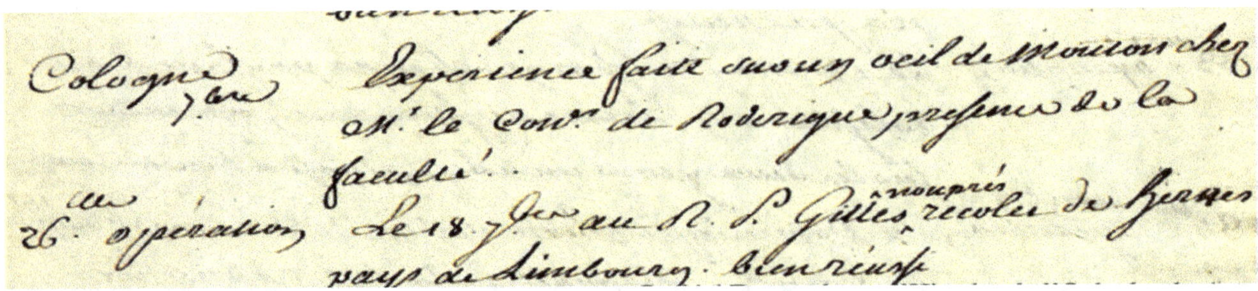

Fig. 19. Daviel's unpublished log lists the cataract extraction performed in Cologne in Gilles Noupres of Limbourg (Liège) on September 18, 1750.

The notice of September 30, 1750, reads as follows:

The French oculist, Daviel, who is currently operating in Cölln, surpasses all of his colleagues in a certain way that he does not press down the cataracts with a round or flat needle like others do, but pulls them completely out of the globe, and takes away that *corpus mortuum* without the eye suffering the slightest damage. He proved a true and happy trial on a Franciscan Father of Liège, Egydius Nouprez, and put his cataract into the hands of the doctors who were present at the operation.[169]

Daviel's unpublished log indicates that the surgery was performed in Cologne on September 18 on Gilles Noupres *de Herves pays de Limbourg, bien reussi* (Fig. 19). As Aegidus is the Latin form of the name Gilles, it seems the patient's name was Gilles Nouprez. About this surgery, Daviel wrote: "One that I did at Cologne on a monk [*un Religieux*] was an even more striking success as the cataract was soft like jelly. However, the monk was in a state to say the Mass 15 days after the operation." This surgery in Father Gilles Nouprez of Liège on September 18, 1750, is the earliest primary planned extraction of a cataract from the posterior chamber through an incision that has been identified in the history of ophthalmology.

From Cologne, Daviel moved on to Mannheim. According to the Regensberg newspapers, he had been in Mannheim since October 22 and would be expected to remain there until November 20, 1750. The newspaper reported: "There [in Mannheim], he has already pulled various cataracts completely out of the eye according to his new method" (*Er hat daselbst schon verschiedene Staare nach seiner neuen Art völlig aus den Augen gezogen*) (Fig. 20).[170]

---

169 Staats-Relation, vol. 6, 1750, p. 468. "Der Franzosische Oculist, Daviel, so dermalen zu Cölln operiret, übersteiget alle andere seine Collegen in einer gewissen Art, daß er den Staar nicht, wie andere, mit einer runden oder platten Nadel niederdructet, sondern ihn gänzlich aus dem Globo heraus ziehet , und das Corpus mortuum , ohne , daß das Auge den geringsten Schaden leidet , wegnimmt. Er hat eine wahre und glückliche Probe an einem Pater Franciscaner von Luttich, Egydius Nouprez, erwiesen, und dessen weggenommenen Staar denen der Operation zugegen gewesenen Medicis in die Hände gegeben."

170 No author listed, Kurzgefaßter Regensburgischer 1750.

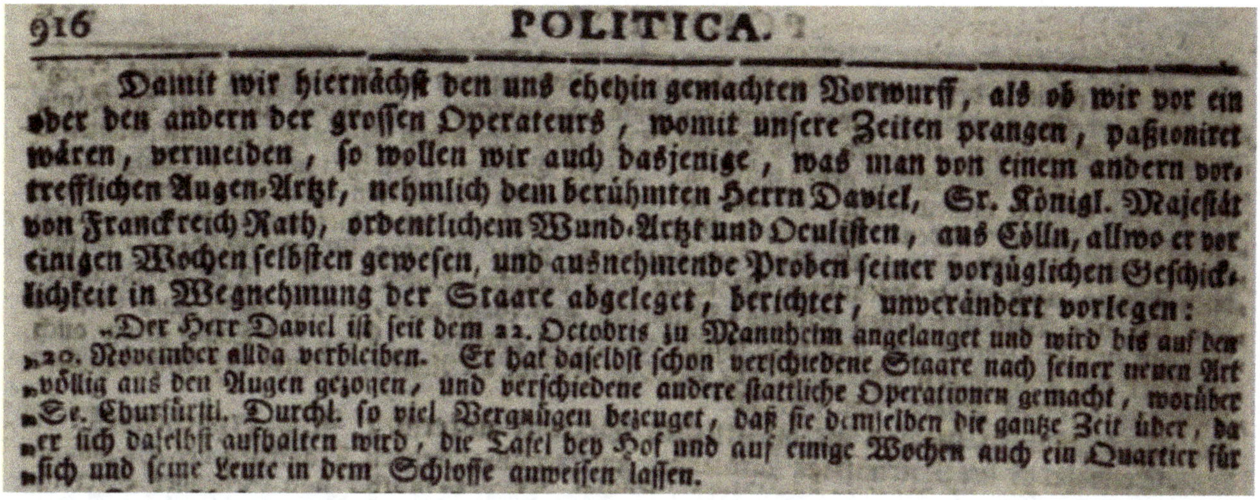

916 POLITICA.

Damit wir hiernächst den uns ehehin gemachten Vorwurff, als ob wir vor ein oder den andern der grossen Operateurs, womit unsere Zeiten prangen, paßioniret wären, vermeiden, so wollen wir auch dasjenige, was man von einem andern vortrefflichen Augen-Artzt, nehmlich dem berühmten Herrn Daviel, Sr. Königl. Majestät von Franckreich Rath, ordentlichem Wund-Artzt und Oculisten, aus Cölln, allwo er vor einigen Wochen selbsten gewesen, und ausnehmende Proben seiner vorzüglichen Geschicklichkeit in Wegnehmung der Staare abgeleget, berichtet, unverändert vorlegen:

„Der Herr Daviel ist seit dem 22. Octobris zu Mannheim angelanget und wird bis auf den „20. November allda verbleiben. Er hat daselbst schon verschiedene Staare nach seiner neuen Art „völlig aus den Augen gezogen, und verschiedene andere stattliche Operationen gemacht, worüber „Se. Churfürstl. Durchl. so viel Vergnügen bezeuget, daß sie demselben die gantze Zeit über, da „er sich daselbst aufhalten wird, die Tafel bey Hof und auf einige Wochen auch ein Quartier für „sich und seine Leute in dem Schlosse anweisen lassen.

Fig. 20. The Regensburg newspaper *Staats-Relation der neuesten europäischen Nachrichten und Begebenheiten* of November 20, 1750, announced that Daviel is performing cataract extraction in Mannheim according to his new method.

Daviel's unpublished log lists cataract extractions in four patients in Mannheim, performed on October 19, November 5, and (in two patients) on November 21, 1750.[171]

We know more specifics about Daviel's trip to Mannheim based on his surgical colleague Vermale. Daviel arrived in Mannheim and examined "Mr. le Baron de Sikingen, ancient grand Chambellan de S. A. S. Electorale Palatine," who was over 70 years old.[172] Sikingen had had couching performed in one eye, initially in May 1746 by an unknown surgeon. A repeat operation was performed in the same eye by Hilmer on December 28, 1746, because the lens had returned to the visual axis.[173] For the next 3 years, Sikingen could read the Gazettes with the help of *lunettes*.[174] Beginning in April 1750, Sikingen had an *ophtalmie* (inflammation) in the eye that Vermale attributed to the lens dislocating into the anterior chamber.[175] Upon his arrival in Mannheim, Daviel examined the eye and successfully performed *l'extraction* on Sikingen the next day, on October 19, 1750.[176]

Vermale also reported that he had seen Daviel perform cataract extraction from the "second chamber of the aqueous humor" in Mr. Schelemmer, Sécrétaire des Fiefs, age 60 years, on this Mannheim trip. An undated manuscript by Daviel, which logs his cataract extractions between 1745 and 1752, lists Mr. Schelemmer's surgery as taking place November 5, 1750, and as the 28th extraction, right after

---

171 Andre, Daviel 2005.

172 Vermale 1751, p. 13.

173 Vermale 1751, p. 9.

174 Vermale 1751, p. 9.

175 "… le cristallin qui avoit passé dans la chambre antérieure de l'humeur acqueuse…" (Vermale 1751, pp. 18–19)

176 Vermale 1751, p. 19.

the 27th case of Sikingen and before the 29th case of the Baron de Beck, both done in Mannheim in the fall of 1750.[177] To open the eye of Schelemmer, Daviel made "l'incision oblique."[178] This is interesting because Daviel's later inferior corneal incisions would not be described as "oblique." We are not told the size of the incision, or what tools were used to make the incision or to remove the lens. The body ("corps") was delivered "tout entier" without having any imprint from the instrument that opened the capsule.[179] The operation was witnessed by Vermale and by M. Walk, Medecin de la Cours, and three others. Daviel extracted the crystalline lens from the contralateral eye several days later.[180]

On November 21, 1750, Daviel performed two additional cataract extractions in Mannheim, in the presence of Vermale and several other named witnesses. Daviel performed *l'extraction* on the 57-year-old Mr. le Baron de Beck, Ecuyer de son Prince.[181] The same day, Daviel also extracted the cataract on the 29-year-old Henri-Francois Kerthenayer, garcon Tailleur & Tambour ... de Heidelberg.[182] In none of the four cases Vermale described did he indicate the size of the incision, whether scissors were used, or the tool used to enter the eye.

Vermale called Daviel's method new and indicated that Daviel had only recently been performing the surgery: ... *la nouvelle méthode que ce fameux Oculiste a imaginé & mis depuis peu en pratique avec beaucoup de succès*). In fact, Vermale specified that Daviel had only performed the procedure 23 times: ... *dans vingt-trois extractions qu'il a déja fait, aucun mauvais succès ne la point encore mortifié*.[183] According to Daviel's unpublished log, if the final Mannheim patient's cataract was the 23rd to be extracted, then the first cataract extracted (factoring in the five bilateral cases) would have been in the 80-year-old widow operated in Auxerre, sometime in the last 4 months of 1749.[184] But there is a really fascinating correspondence between Vermale's figures and Daviel's later unpublished manuscript, which numbers by the patient rather than the operated eye. The final Mannheim patient, Kerthenayer, was later listed as the *30me opération* of extraction performed by Daviel.[185] If Kerthenayer were actually the 23rd patient, in accord with Vermale's letter, then the first cataract extraction would actually be the one listed as *8me opération*, performed on August

---

177 André, Daviel 2005. For some reason, Vermale (1751, p. 30) listed Schelemmer's surgery as May 5, 1748 rather than Nov. 5, 1750. It is possible that Vermale made a mistake, or that his handwriting was difficult for the printer to interpret. But Vermale is describing Daviel's trip to Mannheim in the autumn of 1750, and lists the surgery in the same order as Daviel (2004), i.e. between the 1750 surgeries of Sikingen and the Baron de Beck.

178 Vermale 1751, p. 30.

179 Vermale 1751, p. 31.

180 Vermale 1751, pp. 29–35.

181 Vermale 1751, pp. 35–36.

182 Vermale 1751, pp. 39–42.

183 Vermale 1751, p. 5.

184 Daviel, Andre 2004.

185 Daviel, Andre 2005.

17, 1749.[186] Of note, Daviel's manuscript has, before this operation, and the case of the wig-maker Garion, labeled the *7me opération* on April 6, 1747, one additional unnumbered case of extraction on July 29, 1749, which he must have remembered after preparing an initial draft of his list.[187] Thus, if we accept Vermale's count of 23 cases, Daviel's first extraction could be no earlier than the summer of 1749.

While on this trip to Mannheim, at the age of 54 years, Jacques Daviel made a fateful decision, which transformed ophthalmology:

> During the following three years, I practised this operation [cataract extraction] *quelquefois* [sometimes] on living subjects, to accustom myself to it. But it was only in the course of a voyage that I made at Mannheim in order to treat Son Altesse Serenissime, Madame la Princesse Palatine de Deux Ponts, who had an ancient illness in her left eye that I took the resolution henceforth no longer to operate on the cataract but by extraction of the lens.[188]

The letter of Raimon de Vermale describing Daviel's cataract extractions in Mannheim was written on November 25, 1750,[189] and was apparently published in Paris between January and March 1751.[190]

Were there parallels between Pallucci's case and Daviel's subsequent decision to perform cataract extraction? Pallucci certainly thought so. He wrote in a work that was approved by M. Morand and M. Bourdelin of the Académie Royale des Sciences on September 4, 1751 (Fig. 21):

> Before M. Vermale had informed the public of the prodigious cures made by M. Daviel in the Palatinate, by the extraction which he calls new operation, I had applied myself to it for a long time; we can be sure of this, among other things, by the sixth Observation [on the soldier Pagliano] which I gave in a Brochure printed in 1750. Several experiences which I have made give me the facility of speaking about it.[191].

---

186 Daviel, Andre 2004.

187 Daviel, Andre 2004.

188 Daviel, Pearce 1967.

189 Stricker 1899, p. 273. The letter refers to events up through November 25, 1750 (Vermale 1751, p. 37).

190 This dating is based on the fact that the letter was dated 1751. Vermale refers to April of 1750 simply as "le mois d'Avril" (Vermale 1751, p. 19) without feeling the need to distinguish between April 1750 and April 1751. Moreover, Vermale's letter was responded to by M. Van-Sweiten of Vienna in April 1751, and was referred to by Pallucci in a treatise approved on September 4, 1752 (Pallucci "Methode d'abbattre" 1752, p. 157).

191 "Avant que M. Vermale eÛt instruit le Public des cures prodigieuses faite par M. Daviel dans le Palatinat, par l'extraction qu'il appelle nouvelle operation, je m'y étois appliqué despuis long-temps; on peu s'en assurer entre autres par la sixiéme Observation que j'ai donnée dans une Brochure imprimée en 1750. Plusiers expériences que j'ai faites me procurent la facilité d'en parler." (Pallucci "Methode d'abbattre" 1752, p. 157) A footnote explains that by "the Brochure of 1750", he refers to: Pallucci, Histoire de l'operation de la Cataracte ..." 1750.

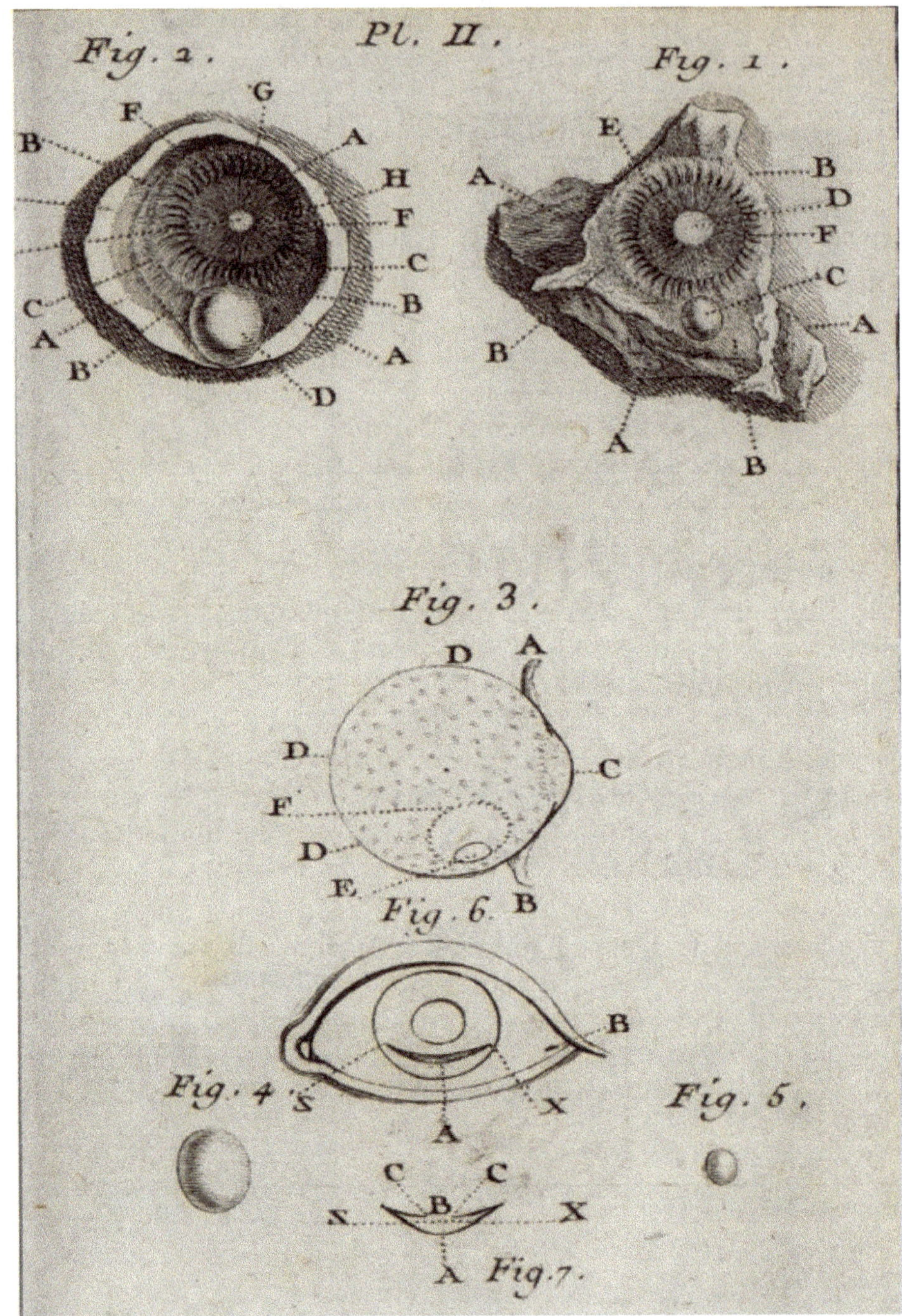

Fig. 21. Pallucci in September 1751 depicted the corneal incision he used for cataract extraction (Pallucci "Methode d'abbatre" 1752, p. 161, Plate II, Fig. 6).

So, with justification or not, Pallucci claims that he has been working on the problem of cataract extraction "for a long time."

In addition, Pallucci suggests in this work approved by the Académie in September 1751, and approved by the censor December 15, 1751, that the incision should be made not with a needle followed by scissors according to "la méthode de M. Daviel," but rather with a single knife: ... *les ciseaux ne sont pas propres pour agrandir l'ouverture de la Cornée* ....[192] Vermale had not even mentioned that Daviel used scissors, or described how Daviel made his incisions. Pallucci must have known about Daviel's method based on informal written or verbal communication among Parisian surgeons, such as Morand. Ironically, Pallucci seems to have published some of the specifics of Daviel's surgery and an improvement on the technique even before Daviel could publish his technique. This September 1751 passage by Pallucci was heralded as being the first to suggest making the incision with a single instrument in an appendix by the Academy of Surgery when Daviel's method was first published in 1753.[193] In reality, Woolhouse had already taught his students the single-knife incision for when the opacified crystalline lens had dislocated into the anterior chamber as early as 1721, and Woolhouse's notes to that effect were published posthumously in 1745.[194] So, the single-knife corneal incision actually predated planned cataract extraction.

From September 15, 1751, to October 5, 1751, Daviel performed 43 cataract extractions while residing in Reims.[195]

On March 14, 1752, a student, M. Thurant, presented to "Les Ecoles de la Faculté de Medecine de Paris" his thesis on cataract extraction, concluding that it was superior to couching. Thurant did not mention Daviel by name, but did mention the cataract extractions Daviel had performed in Reims in the presence of competent doctors and surgeons, who judged that of the 43 cataracts operated, 24 were "perfectly cured,, 9 saw "weakly," and 10 remained "blind."[196] Moreover, Thurant formally presented Daviel's method, involving enlarging the corneal incision with scissors ("ciseaux"), disrupting the capsule with a needle, and then introducing a spatula to deliver the lens.[197] Thurant is the first to explain that gentle pressure is placed upon the eye to deliver the lens in Daviel's method.

Heading into 1752, if you had followed Daviel's letters of 1748 and 1749, Daviel's advertisements, the accounts in the German newspapers, Vermale's letter, Pallucci's writings, and Thurant's thesis, you would have thought that Daviel first performed planned primary cataract extractions in the fall of 1750, shortly after Pallucci's

---

192 Pallucci "Methode d'abbattre" 1752, pp. 159–60, 200–01.
193 Daviel 1753, p. 353.
194 Leffler "Woolhouse" 2017.
195 Delacroix 1890, p. 12.
196 Thurand 1760, p. 88.
197 Thurand 1760, pp. 80–82.

after-cataract extraction of July 3, 1750. But Daviel had a surprise: In 1752, he claimed that he had been performing cataract extractions on and off over the last 7 years, since 1745, and kept it a secret! He was not specific about what year, what city, what specific date, the name of the patient, or the names of any witnesses. And everyone believed Daviel for the next 250 years!

Daviel presented his own work to the Académie de Chirurgie on April 13, 1752, and a brief summary was published in August 1752 but did not provide specifics of the size of the incisions, whether scissors or spatulas were used, and so on.[198]

On May 2, 1752, Daviel wrote in a private letter to Caqué, a physician in Reims, that "Pallucci" was due to pass through that city and would likely enquire about the patients Daviel had operated on in that city. Daviel called Pallucci pitiable ("pitoyable"), said he typically had to couch patients two or three times, and asked that the sick not be entrusted to Pallucci.[199]

On May 26, 1752, Daviel thanked Caqué for showing Pallucci the patients Daviel had operated on in Reims. Daviel continued:

> the Sr Palluchi has convinced himself that he has published the most beautiful book in the world, though it is of absolutely no use at all; it is not I who condemns him, but the public; you would come to the same conclusion if you had read the book, though it was not he who wrote it in spite of the fact that it appeared under his name. It is his adopted work, he would have better done never to have let it appear. This book expresses poor opinions about my method.[200]

Thomas Hope of England witnessed Daviel perform two cataract extractions in 1752, at some point before September 25. Hope wrote that Daviel "was the first, who, in 1745, began to put it [extraction] in practice."[201] Presumably, Daviel provided that date to Hope. Hope also wrote that Daviel had presented his work to "the Academy of Sciences" (rather than the Académie de Chirurgie), describing "115 surgeries, 100 of which have succeeded." This statement has perplexed historians, who have found no other mention of a presentation at the Academy of Sciences. Hope provides no specifics and does not say he witnessed the presentation. Daviel had presented at the Académie de Chirurgie, whereas Pallucci had discussed cataract extraction, citing Daviel by name, in front of the Académie des Sciences. It seems likely that Hope simply made a misstatement.

---

198 No author listed. Mercure de France, August 1752, p. 45.

199 Delacroix 1890, p. 57.

200 Hirschberg & Blodi 1984, vol. 3, p. 393; Delacroix 1890, p. 59.

201 Hope 1752. If someone carefully reviews the Andre, Daviel 2004 manuscript to see which cases were bilateral, and therefore, when Daviel was claiming the 115th surgery was performed, one could better estimate when Hope's first letter was written.

When Daviel presented his work to the Académie de Chirurgie a second time, on November 16, 1752, he indicated that he had performed 206 cataract extractions, of which 182 were successful (Daviel, Pearce 1967). There were some unusual aspects of the way Daviel recounted his personal path toward cataract extraction. Daviel goes to great lengths to insist he began performing extractions before Pallucci's arrival in Paris, even though the written records do not support the claim.

When in 1748, Daviel first wrote about the 1745 case of the hermit treated in Marseille, Daviel had described it merely as a difficult bilateral couching, which resulted in suppuration and loss of the second eye.[202] But, in 1752, Daviel added that after the couching, he incised the cornea with a needle and scissors to remove blood and lens fragments from the anterior chamber.[203] Hirschberg believed that Daviel misremembered the facts in the second telling: "Daviel apparently transferred in 1752 something that he had experienced at a later operation due to a slip of memory to the operation on the *eremite* [hermit]."[204] By the time of his manuscript running through the end of the 1752, this April 1745 couching of Frere Félix is placed on the list of extractions of cataracts from the posterior chamber, with the outcome *bien reussi*.[205]

In 1752, Daviel claims that after the 1745 case of the hermit, Daviel performed planned cataract extraction from the posterior chamber in five unnamed, undated, and unwitnessed patients with success, but then less fortunate outcomes caused him to abandon extraction and to instead perform cataract couching by a new method with two instruments.[206] From Daviel's 1748 letter, we know that the seventh patient having this new couching technique traveled from Paris to Marseille, arriving in September 1745, and had his cataract couched on October 18, 1745.[207] If you believe Daviel's 1752 presentation, Daviel had, in October 1745, three options he could have presented for the patient: the old couching technique, the new couching technique, or extraction. By an amazing coincidence, this patient, if he had opted for extraction, would have been the seventh one having extraction, according to Daviel's manuscript discovered in 2004.[208] But, as it happened, the patient made a different choice and became the seventh patient having Daviel's new couching method, according to Daviel's 1748 letter.[209] Clearly, Daviel is conflating his later extraction method with his 1745 couching technique. If you accept all of Daviel's writings uncritically, you would believe he performed five successful cataract extractions between May 5, 1745, and September 4, 1745, and then squeezed in an unknown number of less successful cataract extractions immediately (which strangely

---

202 Daviel 1748; Hirschberg & Blodi 1984, vol. 3, p. 159.

203 Daviel, Pearce 1967.

204 Hirschberg & Blodi 1984, vol. 3, p. 163.

205 Daviel, Andre 2004.

206 Daviel, Pearce 1967.

207 Daviel Sep. 1748.

208 Andre, Daviel 2005.

209 Daviel Sep. 1748.

do not appear in his undated log), and six of the new cataract technique surgeries in a couple of weeks, so that when the patient arrived later in September, he could be the seventh patient to be couched in the new manner.[210] You would also believe that Daviel performed five consecutive successful planned extractions of cataracts from the posterior chamber in mid-1745, but refused to mention that fact in his letters touting his cataract surgery accomplishments and innovations in 1748 and 1749. One might also wonder why he never published the names, dates, or witnesses of these surgeries, or even the city or the year in which they were conducted (Were they in Marseille, or on one of his sojourns to Aix-en-Provence? Were they in 1745 or 1746?). One might also wonder why he was so excited by the prospects of cataract extraction after his experience removing cataract fragments following the failed couching in M. Garion, the wig-maker, which had taken place in Paris by September 1748. The wig-maker's case would have been a setback to what he had supposedly already accomplished. A straightforward reading of Daviel's letters of September 1748 and July 1749 makes it abundantly clear that (with the exception of Garion's case) Daviel was couching, not performing extraction, before July 1749.

This brings us to an analysis of the surgery of M. Garion, the wig-maker. When Daviel initially presented the case in September 1748 and July 1749, he repeatedly referred to it simply as the case of Garion, without specifying the date of the surgery. In 1752, Daviel recounted the tale of an apparently similar surgery in an unnamed patient in whom Daviel performed a failed couching, followed by a corneal incision, and then extraction of lens fragments from the posterior chamber.[211] This patient has generally been assumed to be same as the wig-maker Garion, whom Daviel had written about since September 1748. But in his 1752 report, Daviel specifies that the patient was operated on April 8, 1747, that is, just before Pallucci arrived in Paris. And Daviel's undated manuscript confirms that Daviel was claiming he operated on Garion on April 8, 1747.[212] By not providing Garion's name in 1752, Daviel prevented anyone from confirming with Garion whether he really had the surgery before Pallucci arrived in Paris. Whereas previously Daviel had not stated how he performed the incision, now Daviel specified that it was made by introducing a needle and then enlarging the incision with scissors ("des petits ciseaux courbes").[213] In 1748, Daviel had specified that a needle (*aiguille*) was introduced into the eye to remove the cataract. In the 1752 version, the incision was so large that Daviel was able to introduce a small spatula (*ma petite spatule*).[214] In 1748, Daviel just indicated that the crystalline was extracted, but in 1752, he clarifies that the lens had been broken into fragments, which were extracted.

---

210 Andre, Daviel 2005; Daviel Sep. 1748.

211 Daviel, Pearce 1967.

212 Andre, Daviel 2005.

213 Daviel 1753, pp. 339, 343; Daviel, Pearce 1967.

214 Daviel 1753, p. 343.

In summary, Daviel in 1752 suggests that the size of the incision, and his manner of making the corneal incision with a needle followed by scissors, has not evolved at all since an initial attempt in 1745.

There is a tell-tale clue that the cases of Garion and all those before him were not the cataract extractions, which Daviel ultimately pioneered in 1750: When Daviel recounts these earlier experiences in detail, he never indicates that he presses on the eye with the finger, even though that is part of his current protocol.[215]

A straightforward reading of these stories raises difficult questions. Daviel made contemporaneous claims to incising the cornea of Garion to extract the cataract (or its fragments) by September 1748. But when Daviel recounts that era in 1752, he bends over backward to describe multiple instances of this event before Pallucci arrived in Paris in July 1747: the hermit in 1745, the unnamed individual in April 1747, and a handful of other unnamed, undated, and unwitnessed cases in between them. And Daviel does so in ways that are self-contradictory.

Daviel was willing to cite Taylor and Freytag as relevant prior art on the cataract extraction question,[216] as their claims could be dismissed with respect to the lack of witnesses, and specificity about the technique. But Daviel refused to even mention Pallucci's name in any of his publications and condemned him in his private letters. The discussion at the Academy after Daviel's presentation credited Pallucci with proposing the single-knife incision by September 1751,[217] but Daviel did not mention Pallucci.

Summarizing Pallucci and Daviel (1750)

If we tell the story of Daviel and Pallucci using only contemporaneously documented evidence, the matter is simplified. Daviel arrived in Paris in November 1746, and Pallucci arrived there in July 1747. Both surgeons worked with the surgeon Morand to perform or assist with cataract surgeries at the Hôtel Royal des Invalides. Both Daviel and Pallucci saw the limitations of traditional cataract couching and worked to improve cataract surgery. By September 1748, Daviel had a case in which he made a corneal incision big enough to introduce a needle into the eye to remove either the lens or fragments of the lens, following a failed couching, perhaps in a manner similar to that of Freytag a half century earlier. On July 3, 1750, Pallucci made a corneal incision big enough to introduce forceps into the eye to remove opacities from the visual axis following a failed couching and published his experience on September 5, 1750. On September 18, 1750, while in Cologne, Daviel performed a planned, primary cataract extraction on Gilles Nouprez, a Franciscan Father of Liège. This surgery is the earliest identified planned primary extraction of a cataract *in toto*

---

215 Daviel, Pearce 1967.

216 Daviel, Pearce 1967.

217 Daviel 1753, p. 353.

from the posterior chamber. On October 19, 1750, while in Mannheim, Daviel made a corneal incision big enough to extract a lens that had dislocated into the anterior chamber following two failed couchings by other surgeons. On November 5 and again on November 21, 1750, while still in Mannheim, Daviel performed planned extractions of cataracts from the posterior chamber in three patients. Daviel resolved on this 1750 trip to Mannheim to stop performing cataract couching and perform cataract extractions exclusively.

Conclusions

Apparent ancient references to removal of cataracts *in toto* through a limbal incision cannot be definitively established, because the surgeons might have been treating a hypopyon. Such cataract extraction through an incision was occasionally performed in the early 1700s when couching accidentally dislocated the lens into the anterior chamber. Planned cataract extraction became a standard technique after Jacques Daviel performed the technique in September 1750 in Cologne on a Franciscan father, and Daviel presented his method in 1752.

Though never as common as cataract couching, aspiration of cataracts was probably performed occasionally in Greco-Roman antiquity, and throughout the medieval Arabic period. As documented by Evliya Çelebi in 1655, cataract aspiration continued to be performed in the Ottoman Empire in the mid-17th century. In fact, it is conceivable that Çelebi described the surgical technique to Western physicians at the peace talks between the Habsburgs and the Ottomans in Vienna in 1665. Çelebi could conceivably even have spoken with Rocci Mattioli, the Italian surgeon who served the Austrian Habsburgs and was credited with the idea in Europe by 1669. Cataract aspiration was attempted, with occasional success, after Daviel's presentation, as we will see in subsequent chapters.[218] Cataract aspiration became the dominant extraction technique after 1967, when Charles Kelman reported preliminary results in breaking up the cataract by phacoemulsification.[219]

Daviel's planned cataract extraction has typically, and correctly, been viewed as an outgrowth of the practice of extracting the crystalline lens from the anterior chamber after the lens had been placed there in the course of a failed couching. But Daviel's work was also an outgrowth of the tradition to remove the parts of the lens, even from the posterior chamber, by pulling them from the eye. Variations on this technique had been discussed in the literature at least since the 1596 animal work of Durante Scacchi of Italy. Daviel cited Freytag, who may have extracted fragments of an after-cataract from the eye with a hooked needle in the 1690s. Pallucci was another surgeon who pulled residual lens material from the eye, and in fact, Pallucci did so in Paris just weeks before Daviel can be documented to have performed planned cataract extraction in the fall of 1750. Daviel criticized Pallucci's work in

---

218 Laugier 1847; Leffler "Aspiration" 2017.

219 Kelman 1967.

his private letters. In Daviel's publications, he refused to even mention Pallucci's name. Daviel wrote Pallucci out of the history.

Although Daviel's method worked for him, and for some other dedicated oculists, many eye surgeons over the next century continued to perform cataract couching. In the British Isles, only about half of cataract surgeons had adopted cataract extraction by 1800.[220] In the United States, only about one-third of cataract surgeons had adopted extraction by 1800.[221] It was not feasible to suture the incision in Daviel's day. The primary comparative disadvantage of couching was the recurrence of vision loss if the lens floated back into the visual axis. Many surgeons reasoned that they could simply repeat the couching if this occurred. Cataract extraction became a more broadly accessible technique after preoperative pupillary dilation began to be used in the early 1800s, general anesthesia became commonly used in the West in the 1840s, aseptic techniques were understood beginning in the 1860s, and topical anesthesia with cocaine was introduced in 1884.

References

Albucasis, Spink MS, Lewis GL (trans.). *Albucasis on Surgery and Instruments: Abu al-Qasim Khalaf Ibn Abbas al-Zahrawi.* Berkeley: University of California Press; 1973.

'Ammār ibn 'Alī Mawşilī, Meyerhof M. *Las Operaciones de catarata 'e 'Ammar i'n 'Ali al-Mawsili.* Barcelona: Laboratories del Norte de Espana; 1937:52–3.

André L, Daviel J. "Liste des Malades a qui J'ai Fait l'extraction de la Cataracte de la Chambre Postérieure de l'oeil par la nouvelle methode que j'ay inventé a Marseille depuis 1745." Un manuscrit inédit de Jacques Daviel. Par le Médecin Général Inspecteur Louis André. Communication à la Société Francophon' d'Histoire d' l'Ophtalmologie. le 8 mai 2004 à Paris France. Provence historique: Revue Trimestrielle; 2005: 421–33. https://www.snof.org/encyclopedie/un-manuscrit-in%C3%A9dit-de-daviel

Arrachart JN. *Mémoires, dissertations, et observations de chirurgie.* Paris; 1805: 115–116. gallica.bnf.fr

Banister R. *A Treatise of One Hundred and Thirteen Diseases of the Eye.* New York: De Capo Press; 1971: 60–1. (Originally published 1622)

Bilsel Y. *Evliya Celebi's Description of the Removal of a Musket Ball From the Brain of a Habsburg Prince: An Interesting Excerpt From the "Seyahatname".* World J Surg. 2012;36(4):923–7.

Blankaart S. A physical dictionary in which all the terms relating either to anatomy, chirurgery, pharmacy, or chymistry are very accurately expl'in'd, by Stephen Blancard. London: J.D. 1684.

Blankaart S. Nieuwe konst-kamer der chirurgie ofte heel-konst, in welke het pit der gantsche chirurgie, op waarachtige en zekere gronden gebouwd is: Verhandelende van de instrumenten, konstiperationien, verlossen der vrouwen, steen-snijden, breuken, geswellen, sweeren, wonden, been-breuken, ontwrigtingen, spaanse pokken, &c 2nd ed. Amsterdam: Jan ten Hoorn, 1685, p. 64.

Blodi FC, Rademaker WJ, Rademaker G, Wildman KF (trans.), Wafai MZ (ed.). *The Arabian Ophthalmologists.* Compiled from original texts by J. Hirschberg, J. Lippert and E. Mittwoch. Riyadh: King Abdulaziz City for Science and Technology. 1993.

---

220 Leffler "British Isles" 2021.
221 Leffler "1491" 2017.

Çelebi E, Kreutel RF. Im Reiche des goldenen Apfels; des türkischen Weltenbummlers Evliyâ Çelebi denkwürdige Reise in das Giaurenland und in die Stadt und Festung Wien, anno 1665. Graz, Verlag Styria; 1957.

Çelebi E, Dankoff R. Evliya Çelebi in Bitlis: the relevant section of the Seyahatname. Brill; 1990.

Çelebi E, Dankoff R, Kim S. *An Ottoman Traveller: Selections from the 'Book of Travels' of Evliya Çelebi, translation and commentary by Robert Dankoff and Sooyong Kim.* London: Eland; 2010: 242-7.

Chauliac G, Nicaise E (trans.). *La Grand Chirurgie de Guy de Chauliac. Chirurgien, Maistre en Medecine de L'Universite de Montpellier. Composee en l'An 1363.* Paris: Bailliere; 1890.

Cleland A. XXVII. A description of needles made for operations on the eyes, and of some instruments for the ears, by the same. 1740;41 (461): 847–51.

Colombo R. De Ocvlis Liber X. In: De re anatomica libri XV. 1559, p. 219.

Compier AH. Rhazes in the renaissance of Andreas Vesalius. Medical history. 2012;56(1):3–25.

Coulon H. La Communauté des Chirurgiens-Barbiers de Cambrai (1366-1795). J.-B. Baillière et Fils; 1908.

Daviel J. Lettre de M. Daviel, Conseiller, Chirurgien ordinaire du Roi en Survivance & par quartier, à M. de Joyeuse, Docteur en Medecine de l'Université de Montpellier, Aggregé au Collége des Medecins de Marseille, & Médecin des Hôpitaux des Galéres. Mercure de France. Paris. 1748, p. 198–221.

Daviel J. *De Heer Daviel, wonende op de Malaquay-Kade te Pary'.* 's Gravenhaegse courant, 1749, p. 2.

Daviel J. Réponse de M. Daviel, Conseiller-Chirurgien ordinaire, & Oculiste du Roi, à la Lettre Critique de M. Roussilles. Mercure de France, Paris. July 1749; 7: 206–227.

Daviel J. [Gazette d'] Amsterdam: avec privilege de nos seigneurs, les états de Hollande et de West-Frise. Amsterdam; 1750.

Daviel J. Sur une Nouvelle Methode de Guérir la Cataracte par l'Extraction du Crystalllin. Mémoires de l'Académie Royale de Chirurgie, T. II, Paris; 1753, pp. 337–54.

Daviel JA, Pearce WG (trans.). On a new method to cure cataract by extraction of the lens by Jacques Daviel, translated by W. G. Pearce. *Brit. J. Ophthalmol.* 1967;51(7):449–58.

Delacroix H. *Jacques Daviel á Reims.* Paris, Masson; 1890. gallica.bnf.fr

Duddell B. *An appendix to the treatise of the horney-coat of the eye, and the cataract. With an answer to Mr. Chesel'en's appendix, relating to his new operation upon the iris of the eye.* London: E. Howlatt; 1733.

Du Mans R, Schefer C (ed.). Estat de la Perse en 1660, par le P. Raphaël du Mans,...publié avec notes et appendice par Ch. Schefer. Paris: Leroux; 1890, p. 178.

Elgood C. Safavid medical practice; or, the practice of medicine, surgery and gynaecology in Persia between 1500 A.D. and 1750 A.D. London: Luzac, 1970, p. 64.

Fehrenbach J. Une famille de la petite bourgeoisie parisienne de Louis XIV à Louis XVIII: les Gaugé et leurs alliances à travers les archives, 1680-1820. Paris: Editions L'Harmattan; 2007.

Feugère M, Künzl E, Weisser U. Les aiguilles à cataract de Montbellet (Saône-et-Loire). Contribution à l'étude de l'ophtalmologie antique et Islamique. Die starnadeln von Montbellet (Saône-et-Loire). Ein beitrag zur antiken und Islamischen augenheilkunde. Jarbuch des Römisch-Germanischen Zentralmuseums Mainz. 1985;32:24–508.

Feyens T. Thomae Fieni ... Libri chirurgici XII, De praecipuis artis chirurgicae controuersiis: quorum seriem et argumenta sequens pagina exhihet: opeperationuma Hermanni Conringii cura nunc primum edita. Francofurti: Goezium, 1602. p. 30. Hathitrust.org.

Galen, Johnston I, Horsley GHR (trans.). *Method of Medicine, Volume III, Books 10-14. Loeb Classical Library 518.* Cambridge: Harvard University Press; 2011: 536–37.

Garnier M. *The London Monthly Mercury; or, Foreign Literary Intelligencer.* London. Vol. 1; 1753, p. 115.

Gosky LD. *De catarrhacta defendente Leopoldo Dieterico Gosky. – Francofurti.* Zeitlerus; 1695.

Heister L. *A general system of surgery in three parts. Containing the doctrine and management I. Of wounds, fractures, Luxations, Tumours, and Ulcers, of all Kinds. II. Of the several operations performed on all Parts of the Body. III. Of the several bandages applied in all Operations and Disorders ....Translated into English from the Latin of Dr. Laurence Heister* (Vol. 1). London: Innys; 1743.

Helm J. *Die Geschichte der Augenheilkunde in Frankfurt am Main bis zum Beginn des 19. Jahrhunderts.* Johann-Wolfgang-Goethe-Universitaet, Frankfurt am Main; 1965.

Henning A. Zur Augenheilkunde im 18. Jahrhundert: Das «Okulisten-seculum» in Berlin. Fortschritte der Ophthalmologie. 1989;86(3):256–8.

Hirschberg J, Blodi FC (trans.). *The History of Ophthalmology. Volume Two. The Middle Ages; the Sixteenth and Seventeenth Centuries.* Bonn: Wayenborgh Verlag; 1985.

Hirschberg J, Blodi FC. *The History of Ophthalmology. Vol 3. The Renaissance of Ophthalmology in the Eighteenth Century. (Part One) Bonn.* J. P. Wayenborgh Verlag; 1984, pp. 14–229.

Hope T. Extracts of two letters of Thomas Hope, MD to John Clephane, MD, FRS concerning Monsieur Dav'el's method of couching a cataract. *Philoso. Trans Royal Soc London.* 1752;31(47):530–3.

[ibn Sina] Abu Ali al-Husayn ibn Abd Allah ibn Sina (Avicenna), Sardo PA (trans.), Bakhtiar L, Nasr SH (eds.). *The Canon of Medicine (al-Qanun fi'l-tibb) (The Law of Natural Healing). Volume 3. Special Pathologies.* Chicago: Kazi Publications; 2014: 273.

Kelman CD. Phaco-Emulsification and Aspiration: A New Technique of Cataract Removal: A Preliminary Report. *Am J Ophthalmol* 1967;64(1):23–5.

Koch HR, Koch KR. Borri, the Prophet, on "he" Restitutio Humo"um" and on Lens Aspiration in the 17th century/Der Prophet Borri über "ie" Restitutio Humo"um" und die Linsen-Aspiration im 17. Jahrhundert. *Sudhoffs Archiv.* 2017:160–83.

Lascaratos J, Marketos S. The cataract operation in ancient Greece. *Hist Sci Med.* 1982;17(Spec 2): 317–22.

Laugier S. Nouvelle methode d'operer la cataracte, ou Methode par aspiration; par le docteur Laugier, chirurgien de l'hopital Beaujon. Paris: Revue Medico-Chirurgicale de Paris. Tome Premier; 1847, pp. 18–26.

Leffler CT, Schwartz SG, Grzybowski A, Braich PS. The first cataract surgeons in Anglo-America. *Surv Ophthalmol.* 2015;60(1):86–92.

Leffler CT, Hadi TM, Udupa A, Schwartz SG, Schwartz D. A medieval fallacy: the crystalline lens in the center of the eye. *Clin Ophthalmol.* 2016;10:649–62.

Leffler CT, Letocha CE, Pierson K, Schwartz SG. Aspiration of cataract in 1815 in Philadelphia, Pennsylvania. *Dig J Ophthalmol.* 2017;23(4):95.

Leffler CT, Schwartz SG, Wainsztein RD, Pflugrath A, Peterson E. Ophthalmology in North America: Early Stories (1491-1801). *Ophthalmol Eye Dis.* 2017;9:1179172117721902.

Leffler CT, Schwartz SG. A family of early English oculists (1600-1751), with a reappraisal of John Thomas Woolhouse (1664-1733/1734). *Ophthalmol Eye Dis.* 2017 Sep 28;9:1179172117732042.

Leffler CT, Schwartz SG. Hydrophthalmia and paracentesis. In: Leffler CT, *The History of Glaucoma.* Amsterdam: Wayenborgh, Kugler. 2020; pp. 137-51.

Leffler CT, Klebanov A, Samara WA, Grzybowski A. The history of cataract surgery: from couching to phacoemulsification. *Ann Transl Med.* 2020 Nov;8(22).

Leffler CT, Schwartz SG, Peterson E, Couser NL, Salman AR. The first cataract surgeons in the British Isles. *Am J Ophthalmol.* 2021 Oct 1;230:75-122.

Leffler CT. Did Ottoman traveller Evliya Çelebi introduce cataract aspiration into Western Europe in 1665? Researchgate.net. 2022.

Le Grand A, Bome R. An entire body of philosophy according to the principles of the famous Renate Des Cartes in three books (written originally in Latin by the learned Anthony Le Grand). London: Samuel Roycroft. 1694; p. 211.

Lenth B. Bach and the English oculist. *Music Lett.* 1938 Apr 1:182-98.

Lind LR. *Studies in Pre-Vesalian Anatomy: Biography, Translations, Documents.* Philadelphia: American Philosophical Society; 1975.

Lindeboom GA. De oogoperatie op Johann Sebastiaan Bach en diens operateur chevalier John Taylor. *Ned. Tijdschr. Geneesk.* 1985;129:2458-62.

Livingston JW. Evliya Celebi on surgical operations in Vienna. Al-Abhath. 1970;23:225-40.

Malgaigne M. Nouvelles recherches historiques sur la methode par succion pour l'operation de la cataracte. In *Revue Medico-Chirurgicale de Paris.* Paris: Tome Premier. 1847; pp. 187-92.

Marra M, Borriello C (trans.). Giuseppe Francesco Borri, tperatiolli e Salamandre [Giuseppe Francesco Borri, between Crucibles and Salamanders]. 2022. Available from: http://www.levity.com/alchemy/borri_english.htm Accessed March 13, 2022.

Méry J. Œuvres complètes (anatomie, physiologie, chirurgie) de Jean Méry réunies et publiées par le Dr Louis-Henri Petit. Paris: Félix Alcan éditeur. 1888; pp. 540-1. Gallica.bnf.fr

Meyerhof M' L'operation de la cataracte du Chirurgien Antyll' d'Alexandrie. In: Koumaris J (ed.). Livr' d'or a' l'occasion de vingt-cinq an' d'activité chirurgicale du docteur Théodore L. Papayoannou ... Le Caire, le 8 mai 1932. Naumburg-Saale: Lippert & Co. 1932; pp. 115-9.

Muralt J von. Schrifften von der Wund-Artzney. Thurneysen, 1711.

Kurzgefaßter Regensburgischer historischer Nachrichten zum Behuf der neuern europäischen Begebenheiten ... Stück auf das Jahr. Regensburg: Seiffart. 1750; p. 916.

Staats-Relation Der neuesten Europäischen Nachrichten und Begebenheiten, Worinnen das merckwürdigste in Politischen- und Kriegs-Sachen ... vorgetragen, nebst Beylagen und Monathlichen Zugaben (etc.), Volume 6. Regensburg: Seiffart. 1750; p. 468.

Mercure de France. Séance Publique. De l'Academie Royal de Chirurgie, tenue le Jeudi 13 Avril 1752. Mercure de France, 1752, August; 198:45-67.

Pallucci NG. Description d'un nouvel instrument propre à abaisser la cataracte. Avec tout le succès possible. Paris; 1750.

Pallucci NG. Histoire de l'operation de la cataracte, faite à six soldats invalides: pour servier de suite à la description de son nouvel instrument. Paris: Houry; 1750.

Pallucci NG. Nouvelles remarques sur la lithotomie suivies de plusieurs observations sur la separation du penis et su' l'amputation des mammelles; avec figures. Paris: Cavelier; 1750.

Pallucci NG. Lettre a Monsieur le marquis de—sur les opérations de la cataracte, faites par M. Pallucci. Paris: Houry; 1751.

Pallucci NG. Methode d'abbattre la cataracte: dédiée à Madame la Princesse De Conty. Paris: Houry; 1752.

Pérez-Cambrodí RJ, Ascaso FJ, Diab F, Alzamora-Rodríguez A, Grzybowski A. Hollow needle cataract aspiration in antiquity. *Acta ophthalmologica.* 2015 Dec;93(8):782-4.

Philippa M, Debrabandere F, Quak A, Schoonheim T, van der Sijs N. Etymologisch Woordenboek van het Nederlands, Amsterdam: 2003-2009.

[Rhazes] Abū Bakr Muḥammad ibn Zakarīyā Rāzī, Faraj ben Salim (trans.). Continens Rasis. Venice: Johannes Hamman. 1529:41. Available from: https://www.wdl.org/en/item/9553/view/1/102/ Accessed January 20, 2020.

Rotta S. Borri, Franz Joseph. Dizionario Biografico degli Italiani. 1971. Vol. 13. Available from: https://www.treccani.it/enciclopedia/francesco-giuseppe-borri_(Dizionario-Biografico)/ Accessed March 13, 2022.

Saint-Yves C, Stockton J (translator). *A new treatise of the diseases of the eyes. Containing proper remedies, and describing the chirurgical operations requisite for their cures.* London: Society of Booksellers. 1741:231-2.

Savage-Smith E. The practice of surgery in Islamic lands: myth and reality. *Soc Hist Med.* 2000 Dec 1;13(2):307-21.

Savage-Smith E. Ammar ibn Ali al-Mawsili. *Encycopaedia of Islam.* Three. 2008, vol. 2, pp. 92-3.

Savage-Smith E. Could Medieval Islamic Oculists Remove Cataracts? The views of a fourteenth-century Egyptian sceptic. Suhayl. *Int J Hist Exact Nat Sci Islamic Civil.* 2022 Dec 21:7-41.

Scacchi D. Subsidium medicinae, in quo, quantum docta manus praestet ad immanes morbos evellendos mirum in modum elucescit. Apud Bartholomaeum & Simonem Ragusios fratres, Urbini, 1596.

Schröder PH. *Van Aalmoes tot Zwijntjesjager.* Baarn: 1980.

Scultetus J, Lamzweerde JB, Borri GF. Appendix, Variorum tam veterum, quam recenter inventorum Instrumentorum Ad Armamentarium Chirurgicum Joannis Sculteti, Una cum quatuor & centum Observationibus Chirurgicis, Ab expertis hujus faeculi & patriae Practicis annotatis, & collectis Opera & Studio Joannis Baptistae a Lamzweerde, Phil. & Med. Doct. Amstelodami. Someren. 1671.

Shadhilī, Sadaqah ibn Ibrāhīm al-Misrī (14th century). al-'Umdah al-kuhlīyah fī al-amrād al-basarīyah. Bethesda, National Library of Medicine, NLM Unique ID: 9107287. MS. A29.1, pp. 118a-120b.

Shastid TH. Daviel, Jacques. In: Wood CA (ed.). *The American Encyclopedia and Dictionary of Ophthalmology.* Volume V. Chicago: Cleveland Press. 1914; pp. 3751-3777.

Shastid TH. Pallucci, Natalis Giuseppe. In: Wood CA (ed.). *The American Encyclopedia and Dictionary of Ophthalmology.* Chicago: Cleveland Press. 1918; Vol. 12, p. 9215.

Stricker L. *The Crystalline Lens System: Its Embryology, Anatomy, Physiological Chemistry, Physiology, Pathology, Diseases, Treatment, Operations and After-changes with a Consideration of Aphakia.* 1899.

Thurand [Thurant]. Question Medico-Chirurgicale, soutenue dans les Ecoles de la Faculte de Medecine de Paris, le 14 Mars 1752, par M. Thurand … La Methode de guerir la Cataracte par l'extraction du crystallin. In: von Haller A (ed.) Collection de theses medico-chirurgicales: sur les points les plus importants de la Chirurgie théorique & pratique. Paris, Vincet. 1760; pp. 75-88.

Truc H, Pansier P, Liard L. Contribution a l'histoire de l'ophthalmologie française: histoire de l'ophthalmologie a l'École de Montpellier du XIIe au XXe siècle. Paris: Maloine, 1907.

Vermale [de Vermalle] R. Lettre de Monsieur Raimon de Vermale, Conseiller d'Etat, & premier Chirurgien de son A. S. Monseigneur l'Electeur Palatin … A Mr. de Chicoyneau. Conseiller d'Etat ordinaire, & premier Medecin du Roi, sur l'extraction de la cataracte hors de la chambre postérieure de l'oeil: Nouvelle opération imagine & perfectionnée par le célébre Mr. Daviel, Conseiller Chirurgien ordinaire & Oculiste du Roi, & de S. A. S. Monseigneur l'Electeur Palatin. 1751; Archive.org

Watson A. Art. V. Continuation of historical and critical remarks on the operations for cataract. By Alexander Watson, MD. *Edin Med Surg J.* 1846;65:57-68.

Woolhouse JT. A treatise of the cataract and glaucoma: in which the specific distinctions of those two diseases, and the existence of membranous cataracts, are clearly demonstrated … Compiled from the dictates of the late learned and ingenious Mr. Woolhouse, as taken from him in writing, by one of his pupils. London: Cooper, 1745; pp. 18-99.

2. Jacques Daviel and the Presentation of Planned Cataract Extraction (1752)

Daniel M. Albert, MD

Introduction

When the noted French surgeon Jacques Daviel (1693-1762) (Fig. 1) presented his method of cataract extraction to the French Academy of Surgery on April 13, 1752, it marked the beginning of a major departure from centuries-old practice. It was the fruit of years spent mastering traditional methods while developing insights into the potential benefits of a more challenging but superior procedure.

By the time the young Daviel had begun his studies to become a surgeon in early eighteenth-century France, previous investigators had discovered much about the anatomy of the eye, the lens, and even the true nature of the cataract. A few cataract

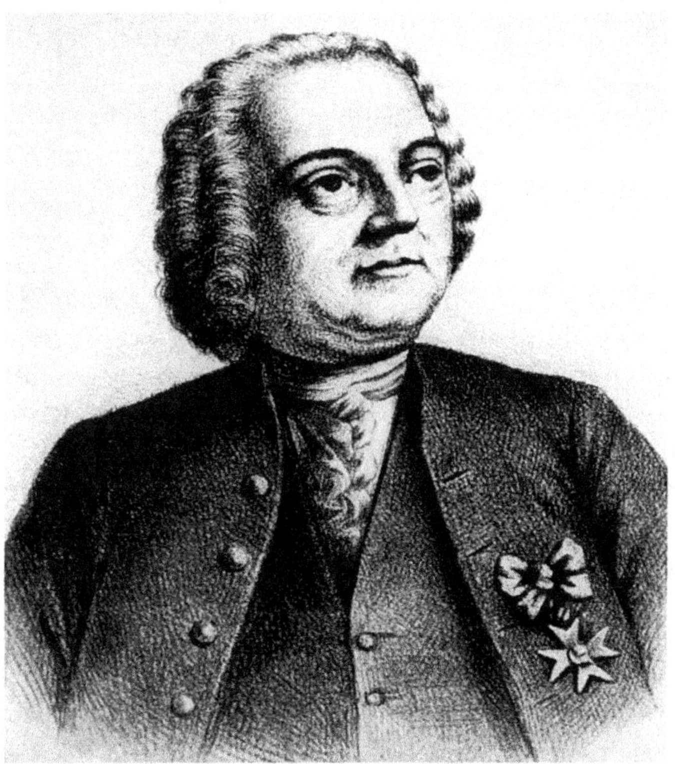

Fig. 1. Jacques Daviel at the height of his fame.
Source: Hirschberg FC. The history of ophthalmology. Vol. 3. Bonn, Wayenborgh, 1984: 150.

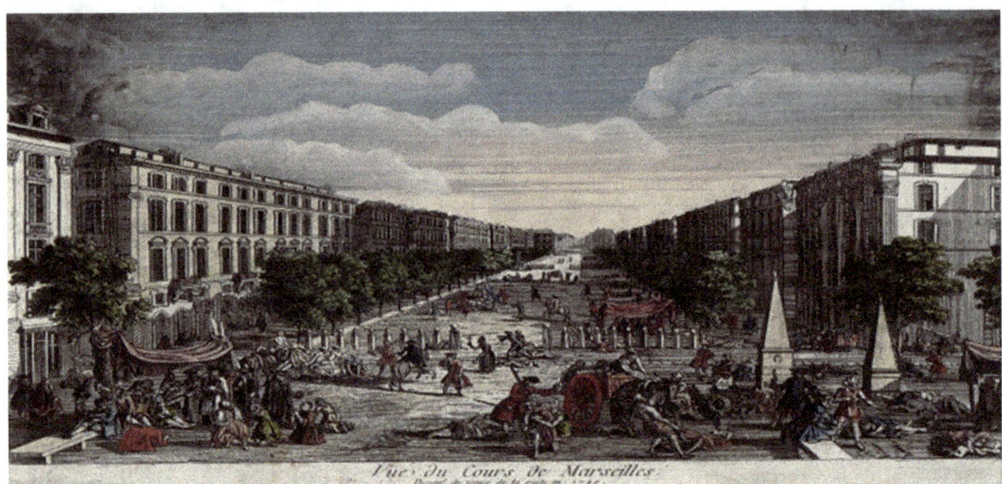

Fig. 2. The main thoroughfare of Marseille during the plague of 1720 by Michel Serre (wellcomeimages.org).

extractions had been reported over the years in different times and places, and more recently a few surgeons had tried, with little success, to champion extraction as a potentially safer advance on the ancient practice of couching. But it was Jacques Daviel, known across much of the European continent as an eye surgeon of exceptional talent, who brought his unique blend of experience, skill, and ingenuity to the task of convincing the world of the value of a new and better approach to dealing with cataracts.

Origins and Early Career as a Surgeon

Daviel was born in August 1693 in La Barre, Normandy. He set his sights early on the life of a surgeon. While still a boy, he reportedly began to form his career aspirations after helping the village surgeon in reducing a man's fractured leg. Although there was no family wealth to support his training, on his father's death he was apprenticed to an uncle, Dr. Sallou, who was a surgeon in Rouen, about 60 miles from Daviel's birthplace. At age 20, he became an assistant surgeon in the French Army, serving in military hospitals and eventually as an assistant to Xavier Bouquot at the Hotel-Dieu in Paris, the only public institution in Paris where cadaver dissection was permitted.

He was still in the army seven years later when Europe's last significant outbreak of bubonic plague struck southern France, claiming the lives of about 100,000 inhabitants of Marseille and its environs before it had run its course[1] (Fig. 2). Daviel responded to news of this scourge by volunteering to join a team of Parisian physicians as an epidemic surgeon to treat plague victims in Salon-de-Provence. With the energetic use of patient isolation and aromatic antiseptics, Daviel served his patients with a level of devotion that earned him the admiration of local residents and, soon after, recognition from France's ruling regency

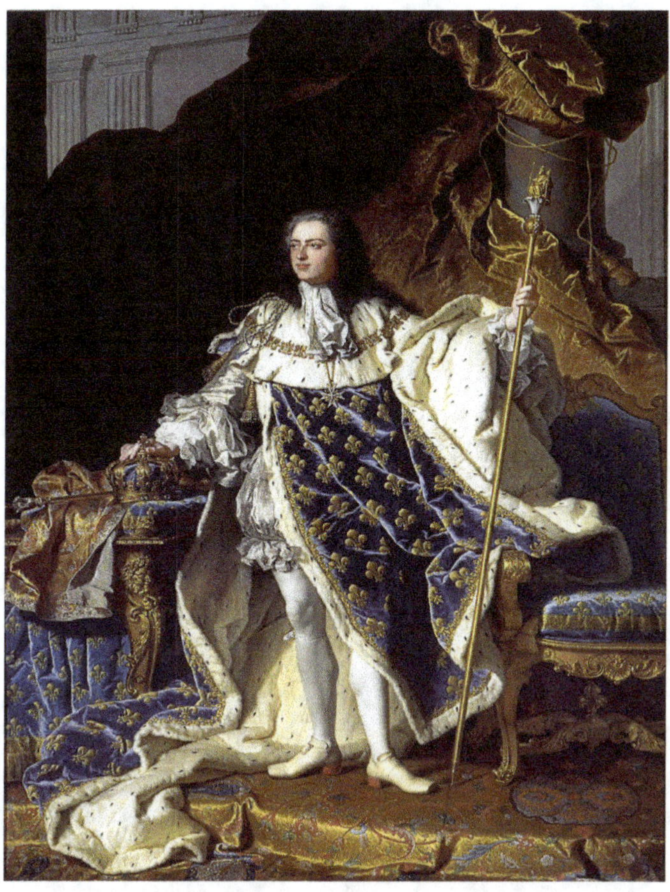

Fig. 3. Portrait of Louis XV of France (1710–1774), the patron and supporter of Daviel, painted by Hyacinthe Rigaud.

(Fig. 3). The city of Marseille awarded him the Cross of Saint Roch (named for the patron saint of the sick), and in 1722 he was promoted to the rank of master surgeon.

When two years after his arrival, he married the daughter of another prominent local master surgeon, the bride's ample dowry offered Daviel an unusual opportunity to pursue his professional goals without a confining sense of financial urgency.[2] Despite having launched his career as a general surgeon, beginning around 1728, it appears that he began to take a particular interest in diseases of the eye.[2]

Couching

At this time, there was one commonly accepted treatment that might succeed in restoring some sight to patients whose vision was obstructed by cataract. For centuries, those who were desperate enough to seek whatever relief was offered for their condition could sometimes find a practitioner of the procedure known as couching. This typically involved the use of a sharp instrument to pierce the eye at the edge

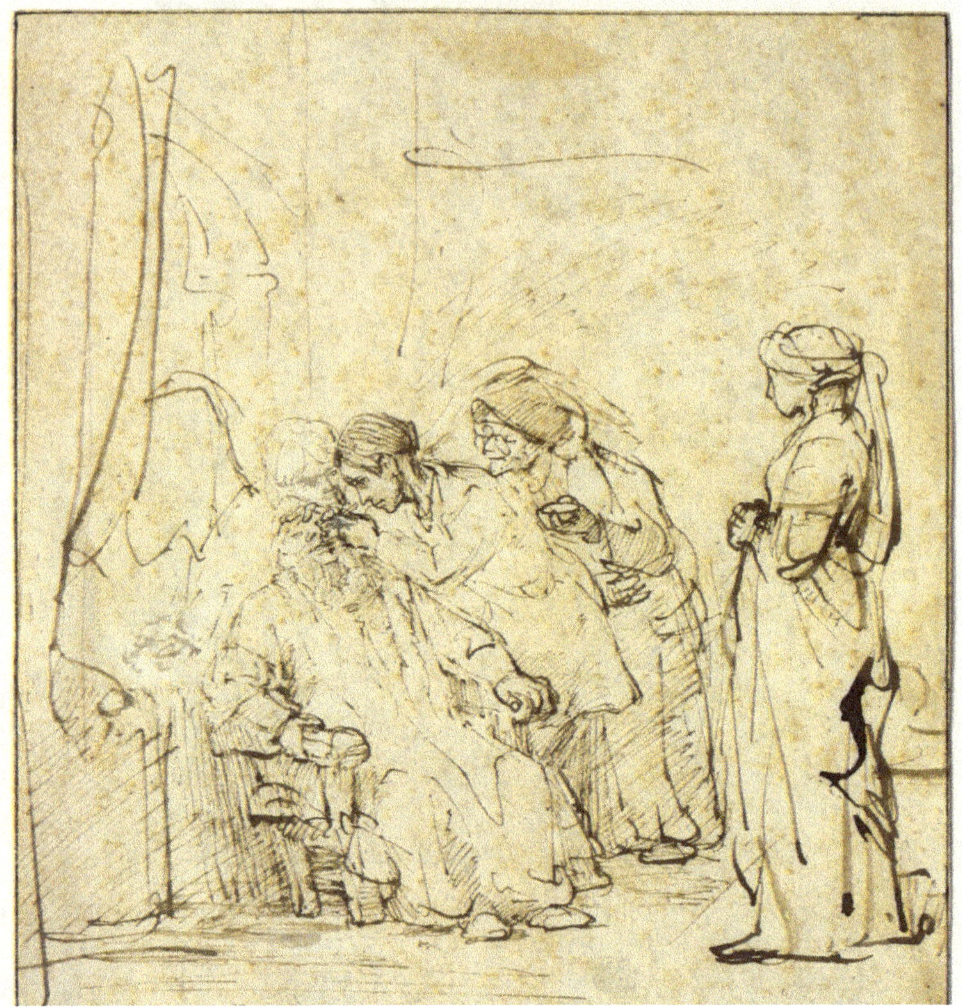

Fig. 4. Rembrandt's depiction of the scene in the Apocrypha in which Tobias, assisted by an angel, heals the blindness of his father Tobit (Cleveland Museum of Art, clemusart.com.).

of the cornea, free the opaque cataract from its position behind the iris, and nudge it into the vitreous compartment where it could no longer block the light passing through the pupil. Despite its often poor outcomes because of infection or its failure to improve vision, couching had been practiced since antiquity (Fig. 4). Other methods were occasionally reported, but couching was still the primary method for treating cataract in Daviel's day.

Daviel Becomes a Cataract Surgeon

Jacques Daviel performed his first couching operation for cataract in 1733 at the age of 40. The procedure was judged a success[3] and likely reinforced Daviel's growing interest in eye diseases. Within a year of this first successful cataract operation, he had decided to specialize in eye surgery (Fig. 5). Biographers have speculated

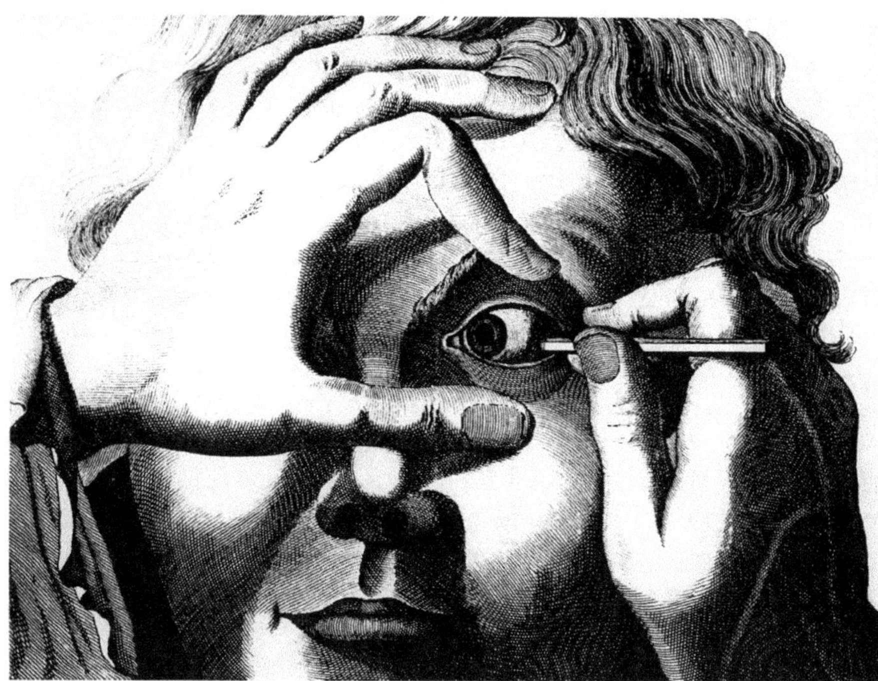

Fig. 5. Contemporary illustration of a couching procedure from the thesis *Animad-versiones de suffusionis natura et curatione* defended by Johann Philipp Schnitzlein under the presidency of Justus Gottfried Günz at Leipzig in 1750 (p. 148).
Source: Hirschberg FC. The history of ophthalmology. Vol. 3. Bonn, Wayenborgh, 1984: 307.

that this decision may have been strongly influenced by his having made the acquaintance of the traveling oculist and self-described "Chevalier," John Taylor, who visited Marseille in 1734. The flamboyant Taylor was eye surgeon to George II, the Pope, and several royal families of Europe, and like many in his profession, he journeyed from town to town performing couching and other procedures on the eyes of patients who had few other options. Taylor, who was perhaps better known for his promotional flair than for his surgical successes, traveled the Continent in a coach painted with images of eyes.[4]

Unlike Taylor, who became notorious for his failures, Daviel soon became highly proficient at couching, which in the days before anesthesia required speed as well as exquisite skills. In the development of these skills, he had the advantage of being able to improve his technique by practicing on cadavers. The reputation he had established with community leaders in Marseille and with the King himself placed Daviel in a position to avoid the limitations on dissecting human bodies that were imposed in many places because of social and religious scruples. Thus, he could make his mistakes and hone his techniques without jeopardizing live patients. (By contrast, his famous contemporary and rival cataract surgeon, Baron Michael Johann Baptist de Wenzel of Lorraine, on being complimented for his dexterity, "acknowledged he had lost a hat-full of eyes before he learned to extract."[5])

From 1734 to 1747, Daviel specialized in couching cataracts, and his reputation in Europe continued to grow. Like his surgeon contemporaries, he traveled to his patients, at first touring through southern France, Spain, and Portugal, and later through Italy, Germany, and Belgium. His progress, and especially his triumphs, while on the road were reported in 29 unsigned articles that appeared in the most widely read newspaper in Provence, the *Courrier D'Avignon*. Biographers attribute these reports to Daviel himself; they gave a detailed accounting of where he was going and when, lodgings where he could be found, how many surgeries he had performed to date, and how many were considered a success. Thus, if someone was emboldened to seek his services, they would know where to find him. In the August 1737 issue of *Courrier d'Avignon*, the anonymous reporter wrote that Daviel "had done over 2000 operations on patients 30, 40, 60 up to 90 years old, among them blind patients between 15 and 54 years of age. He even had the satisfaction of curing several persons, blind since birth, who, after the operation could discern objects shown them". In Spain and Portugal, Daviel was received by the King and the royal family, where he attended members of royalty, aristocrats, and servants.[6]

In 1738, he was elevated to Royal Demonstrator of Anatomy and Surgery at the Hotel-Dieu in Marseille, where he taught public courses in anatomy and surgery (Fig. 6). By 1740, seven years after performing his first cataract surgery, his ability as a coucher had earned him honors that included an appointment as a corresponding member of the Royal Academy in Paris. And in 1746, the 53-year-old Daviel was selected as surgeon-oculist to King Louis XV, whereupon he relocated to Paris. It had been his skill in couching cataracts that contributed most to his success and subsequent honors, but even so, it was at about that time he wrote to a friend that despite his success, he was far from satisfied with the cataract surgery of that day.[3]

Early Discoveries about the Eye and Cataract

Daviel's achievements had been built on the work of many investigators over the course of centuries, beginning with the first recorded ideas about the location and function of the lens and the nature of the mysterious cataract. The neuroanatomist and historian Stephen L. Polyak[7] attributes the first genuine scientific description of the eye to Herophilos (344-280 BCE).[8] The beliefs of other leading scholars from antiquity varied widely. According to Polyak, Hippocrates (460-377 BCE) was unaware that the lens even existed. Aristotle (c. 384-322 BCE) believed that the lens formed post-mortem from an accumulation of phlegm.[9] In the first century AD, Celsus advanced the view that the lens was the vital organ of vision; he described it as consisting of a "humor" or liquid, like an egg white, with an anterior space ("*locus vacuus*") between the front of the lens and the pupil.[10] This concept of the lens and its function became the dominant view for well over a millennium until the Swiss physician Felix Platter (1536-1614) and later the German mathematician and astronomer Johannes Kepler (1571-1630) demonstrated that the structure actually refracted light onto the retina, which was the essential sensitive organ of vision.

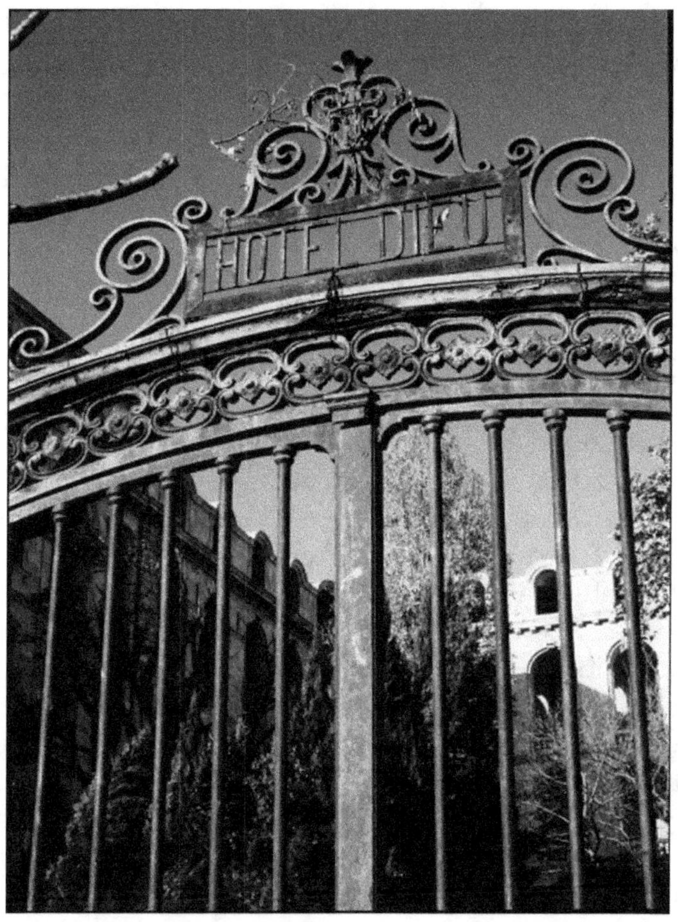

Fig. 6. Entry of Hotel-Dieu in Marseille, photographed by Christophe Moustier.

True Nature of the Cataract Revealed

Regarding the nature of the lens's dark twin, the cataract, the common misconception among physicians of antiquity was that a cataract originated as a humor that flowed into the space between the lens and the pupil, where it solidified into a hardened layer. As a result of this view, according to Daviel,

The ancients who had always considered the cataract as a membrane, devised means of removing it that conformed to their opinions. Some used round needles to roll up this imaginary membrane like a ribbon; others invented extremely pointed needles so as to cause less damage to the sclera; some used cutting needles to sever the threads they believed attached the cataract to the ciliary processes; finally, Freytagius (town surgeon of Zurich) devised a kind of spring forceps terminating in needles, with which he proposed to extract the membranous cataract from the eye.[11]

Not until the seventeenth century was it understood that a cataract was in fact the lens itself, somehow become clouded or opaque. This discovery was reported by Werner Rolfink (1599-1673) in 1656 based on his post-mortem examinations of cataractous lenses and later by Michel Brisseau (1676-1743).[6] In the preface of his book, *Traite de la Cataracte et du Glaucoma* (Paris, Houry, 1709, pp. 38-9), Brisseau recounted the case of a soldier with a cataract who died in 1705. The day after the death, Brisseau couched the cataract, dissected the eye, and removed the lens, revealing to him the cataract's true nature. In 1707, Antoine Maitre Jan (1650-1725) published his own similar findings from examining the lens of a deceased cataract patient in his *Traite des Maladies des Yeux*.

Successful Extractions Demonstrated

During the Middle Ages, Arabian surgeons were aspirating the soft congenital cataract with a hollow needle,[12] but this was an exception; couching remained the principal surgical treatment for cataracts for many years. A generation before Daviel, reports appeared from French surgeons who had tried to remove the lens instead of couching it. In operations by Charles de St. Yves (1667-1736) in 1707 and 1716, and in another by the noted surgeon Jean Louis Petit (1674-1760) in 1708, living patients had lenses subluxed into the anterior chamber. All three procedures were reported to be successful. In 1707, the surgeon Jean Mery (1645-1723) had recommended to the Paris Academy of Science that extraction be recognized by the Academy as a legitimate alternative to couching for treating cataract. According to Mery, "Extraction seems to be as safe as couching; it may be even less risky . . . The aqueous reforms easily. The cornea does not have any blood vessels and therefore does not become affected with inflammations". But the Academy displayed little interest at that time.[13]

Daviel's New Method Evolves

Daviel had read the publications of Brisseau, Maitre Jan, St. Yves, and Petit on cataract extraction. He also knew about Mery's effort to make the case for extraction to the Paris Academy of Science. Daviel's own change of heart on couching versus extraction of cataracts came gradually, and it was based largely on his own experience with the shortcomings of the currently accepted methods. Two of his couching operations were especially influential in changing his thinking.

During a 1745 couching procedure on a Brother Felix, a hermit from Eguilles, the lens broke into pieces as Daviel tried to dislodge it with a sharp needle. Several pieces passed into the anterior chamber, which was soon filled with blood. Daviel stated in 1752 that he was able to open the cornea and remove the lens fragments, following a procedure Petit had described in 1708. In the immediate aftermath, some of Brother Felix's sight in the eye was restored, but it soon became infected and was lost (p. 339).[11]

After this experience, Daviel replaced the customary sharp needles with a blunt instrument of his own design to couch cataracts. Notably, he also resolved at that time to bring a new "great idea" for cataract surgery to a "certainty by continuing to work daily on the eyes of cadavers".[3]

Two years later, on April 8, 1747, Daviel set out to perform a couching operation on the wig maker M. Garion. Daviel's fallback option in response to complications during that operation laid the foundations for his new approach. He later recounted the experience this way:

> I begin with the left eye whose cataract seemed more mature and yet I was not able to depress it. The pupil appeared cloudy after the operation and the patient saw absolutely nothing. I then proceeded to the right eye and had just as much trouble. Having failed in every maneuver to push down the cataract in this eye, I decided to open up the cornea, as I had done with the hermit. I widened the aperture, then I raised the cornea with small forceps, inserted my small spatula through the pupil and extracted from the posterior chamber of the eye the whole lens, divided and broken into several pieces during my initial procedure. After this extraction, a part of the vitreous humor oozed out: it had been disrupted by the first operation but, despite this inconvenience, the patient discerned objects well. The operation had no harmful sequelae and, after some time, the patient was cured.[11, p.343]

This extraction of the cataract of the wig-maker ("*perruquier*") M. Garion performed before September 1748 is considered the first ever documented extraction of a cataract from the posterior chamber (as opposed to the anterior chamber) in the history of ophthalmology. It was not a planned procedure, however. In his letter of September 30, 1748, Daviel wrote, "The observations which I made at this successful operation [on M. Garion] have aroused in me great ideas concerning the extraction of cataract."[15] Nonetheless, all of the other cataract cases performed by Daviel and detailed in his letter of September 1748 were described as cases of couching (*e.g.* "…*j'ai abbattu une cataracte…*").[16]

Even if he did not mention additional extractions in his letter of September 1748, Daviel might have occasionally performed the procedure before 1750 because he reported in 1752:[17]

> "During the following three years, I practised this operation several times on living subjects, to accustom myself to it. But it was only in the course of a voyage that I made at Mannheim in order to treat Son Altesse Serenissime, Madame la Princesse Palatine de Deux Ponts, who had an ancient illness in her left eye that I took the resolution henceforth no longer to operate on the cataract but by extraction of the lens."[18]

This statement dates his routine use of planned cataract extraction, as opposed to couching, to his trip to Mannheim, which is known to have taken place in October 1750 (Fig. 7).[19]

By 1752, Daviel had performed extractions on 206 cataractous eyes, reporting good results in 182 cases, a success rate of 88%. This was in an age when surgery

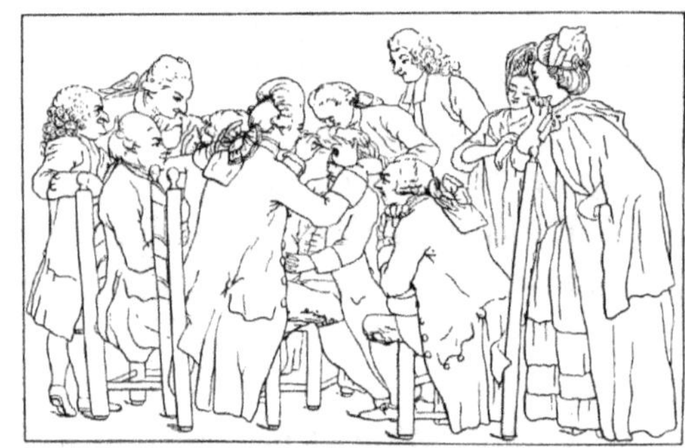

Fig. 7. Baron Wenzel performing cataract extraction on February 4, 1772, in Berlin at the orphanage of the French Colony. This scene was witnessed and then drawn by Daniel Chodowieski (1726-1802) and published in Johann Caspar Lavater's *Physiognomische Fragmente* (1775-8).
Source: Hirschberg FC. The history of ophthalmology. Vol. 4. Wayenborgh. Bonn 1984: 182.

was done without asepsis or anesthesia on patients who were restrained by the surgeon's assistants, and sometimes even bound to a chair. During this time, Daviel continued to refine his techniques, designing new instruments to perform them as he worked with both living patients and cadavers (Fig. 8).

Daviel Describes and Promotes His Extraction Procedure

It was in 1752 that Daviel presented his cataract extraction method to the Royal Academy of Surgery. This was a different and perhaps more practical group than the Academy of Science that had spurned Mery's extraction proposal 45 years before. Following a thorough peer review, Daviel's paper was published in the Academy's proceedings.[11] More than a century later, in an address commemorating the publication of Daviel's landmark 1752 paper, Alvin A. Hubbell presented his translation and summary of the procedure as Daviel had described it:

> The operation which he [Daviel] had invented and now made public consisted in incising the lower part of the cornea exactly at its junction with the sclera. He first made an opening into the anterior chamber at the extreme lower margin of the cornea with a myrtiform or triangular shaped knife, and then, after withdrawing this, he enlarged the incision on both sides with a narrow, blunt pointed, double-edged knife, as far as he easily could and finally when the cornea became too much relaxed to continue the incision he completed it to the extent desired with delicate scissors which were so curved on the flat and edge as to correspond to the curve of the corneo-scleral line. These, of course, were made right and left, and the blade to be introduced into the anterior chamber was blunt pointed. According to his memoir the incision was of equal extent on both sides of the cornea, and was carried to a point

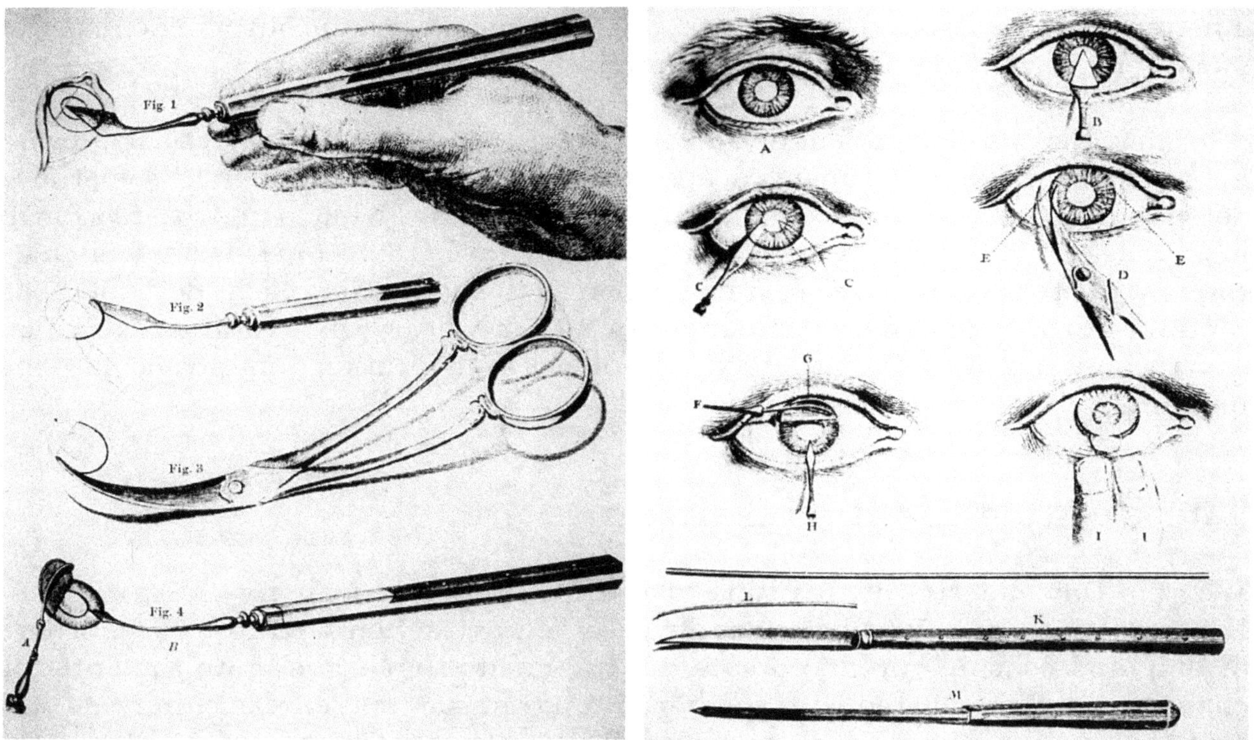

Fig. 8. (a, b) Daviel's cataract extraction technique using the instruments he designed, as presented to the Royal Academy of Surgery April 13, 1752, and published
in the Memoirs of the Royal Academy of Surgery in Paris in 1753.
Source: Hirschberg FC. The history of ophthalmology. Vol. 3. Bonn, Wayenborgh,
1984: 167.

on each side "a little above the pupil." Having completed the incision he gently lifted
up the corneal flap with a small spatula and incised the anterior capsule of the lens
with the sharp-edged needle. After doing this, he carried the spatula between the
lens and the iris, "so as to entirely loosen the cataract and facilitate its issue." After
the cataract was delivered, the corneal flap was then allowed to fall into place. If the
cataract happened to be soft and "glairy" or broken into pieces, the remnants were
removed with a curette. The pupil might sometimes be disarranged by the passage
of the lens, especially if it was large and hard, and it should then be readjusted.
The corneal flap being accurately replaced, the eye was gently cleansed and covered
with a small compress, over which plasters were applied and the whole was kept in
place by a bandage without much pressure.[14]

In reviewing Daviel's proposal, the Academy examined relevant documentation,
identified his patients, and had other surgeons review and attest to their results.
Three surgeons with exceptional credentials performed Daviel's operation during the
following year on 19 elderly soldiers with cataracts at the Hotel Royal des Invalides,
the veterans' hospital in Paris. Of the 38 eyes operated on, 14 had "good vision," 10
had no change, and 14 had reduced vision. Although Daviel himself had reported

a better rate of success, these results were still considered encouraging enough to merit consideration by the surgical community.

From reviewing descriptions of Daviel's cataract extraction procedures, it appears his preferred method was an extracapsular technique. And although he sometimes delivered the lens with its capsule intact, this was not what he advocated for in most cases. The French surgeon Georges De La Faye (1699–1781) is often cited as the first to promote intracapsular extraction as the better approach. Both methods continued to be employed until late in the twentieth century when cataract extraction was revolutionized by the introduction of phacoemulsification and intraocular lens implants.

The Contest for Recognition

Why did Daviel decide at this time to entirely replace couching with extracapsular extraction? He might have simply reserved extraction for those cases where attempts at couching produced cataract fragments that moved into the anterior chamber, as had occurred with the hermit and the wig maker. Couching was still quicker and less painful, especially in the absence of anesthesia. Couching probably also presented less risk of infection with its small corneal opening. Even for Daviel, the visual results from the two procedures were comparable. Given all this, it is reasonable to assume that it was the very novelty and difficulty of extracting, the opportunity to display his surgical skills, and the chance to claim credit as the originator of extraction that motivated him.

Daviel had many competitors for the distinction of having invented the first practical procedure for cataract extraction. Among them were Jean Baptiste Thurant, John Taylor, Georges de La Faye, and Samuel Sharp, as well as others. However, Daviel could claim precedence, and among his colleagues there was little dispute about his good results.

In the years that followed, Daviel actively defended his method of operating on cataracts. By 1756, he had performed 434 cataract extractions, of which 384 were reported to be "perfectly successful. In 1757, Daviel's son Jacques Henri, training as a surgeon in Paris, published his medical thesis describing and explaining the superiority of his father's approach. Yet, until the end of the nineteenth century, surgeons in Europe and England were divided between those who preferred couching and those who preferred extraction—a dispute that medical historians have often termed the "hundred years war" (Fig. 9).

Daviel eventually became an internationally recognized figure and the recipient of many honors, including membership in the Royal Society of London (1756) and the Royal Society of Sweden. Late in his career, he developed a strong curiosity about how congenitally blind persons perceived objects, and he corresponded on

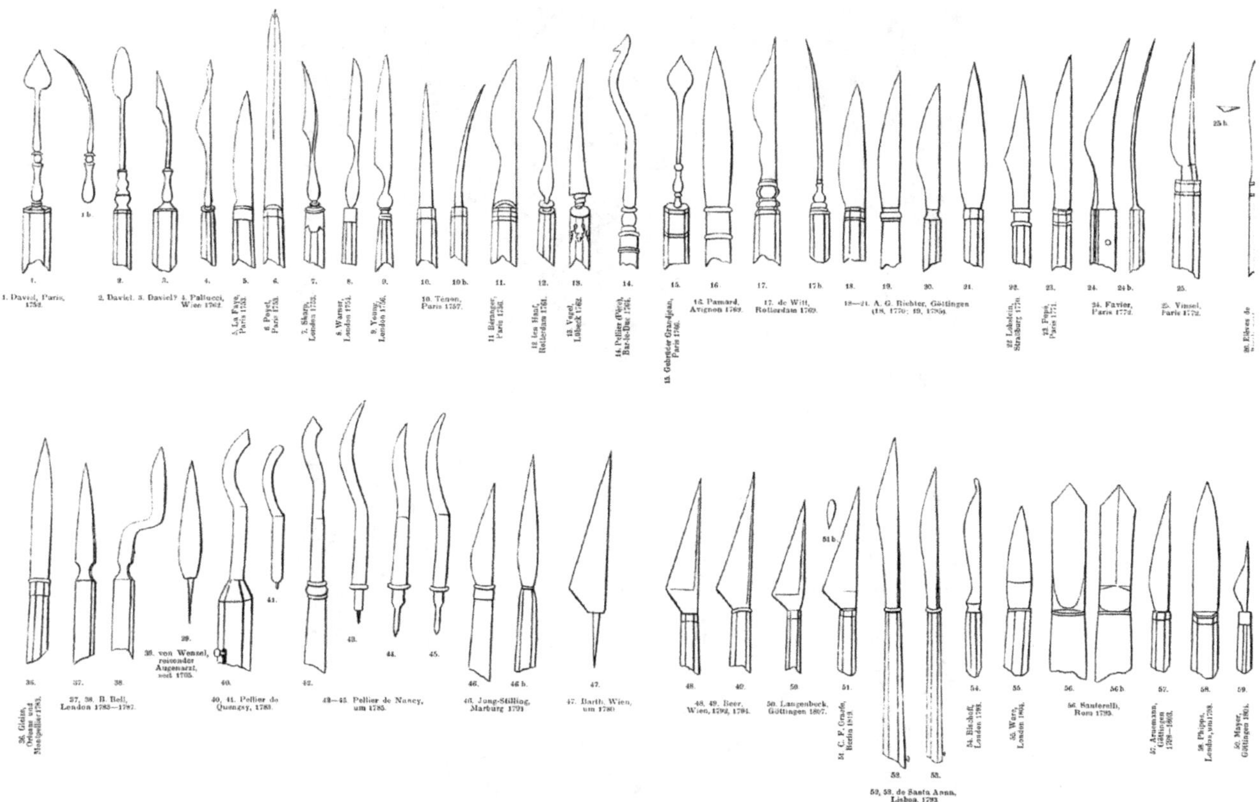

Fig. 9. The cataract knives introduced by Jacques Daviel and his rivals.
Source: Hirschberg FC. The history of ophthalmology. Vol. 3. Bonn, Wayenborgh,
1984: 191.

the subject with the noted Swiss physiologist Albrecht von Haller. His own findings
were based on 22 cases of congenital cataract he had operated on.

Near the end of Daviel's life, Louis XV created a chair of ophthalmology in Paris,
but it was too late for Daviel to fill. In 1762, apparently afflicted by cancer of the
larynx, his health deteriorated and his speech became impaired. A friend had to
read for him his final paper on cataract extraction before the Royal Academy of
Surgeons in April. He died on September 30 of that year (Fig. 10).

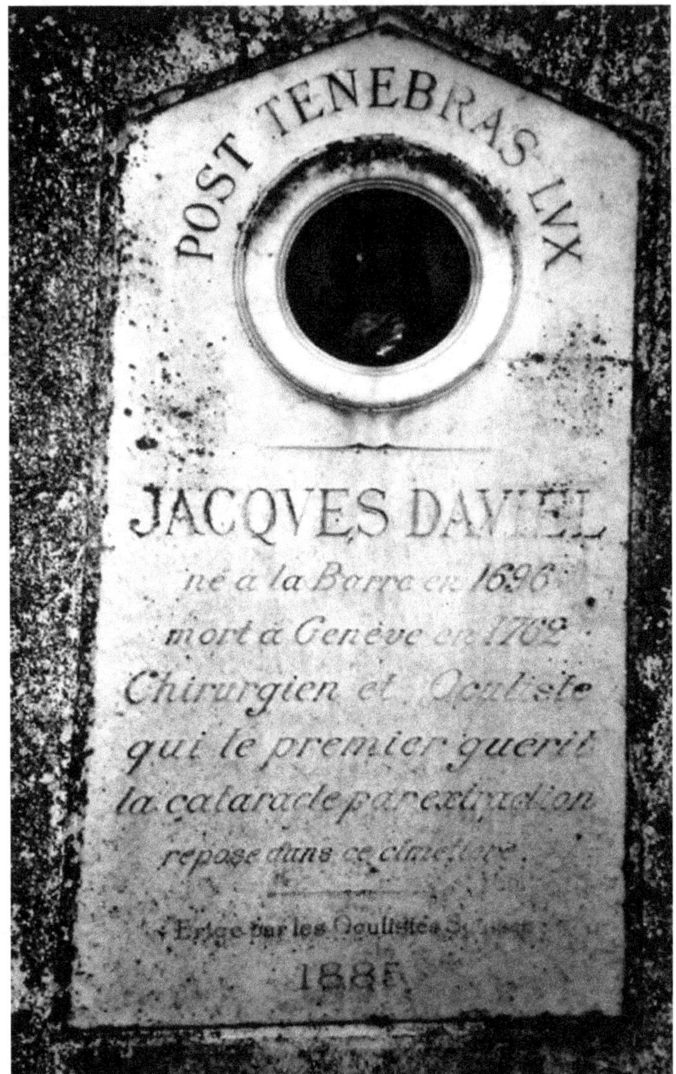

Fig. 10. Tombstone of Jacques Daviel (snof.org).

Conclusion

Jacques Daviel lived in a period when the cataract's true anatomic nature at long last became clear. His general surgical training was the best available at the time, and his access to cadaver material for practice surgery was unique for that age. Daviel's native surgical skills and his gradual focus on the surgery of the eye as his sole specialty combined to qualify him to introduce *cataract extraction,* a revolutionary advance in cataract surgery technique. Moreover, he convinced many leading contemporary surgeons that extraction had advantages over the centuries-old method of couching the cataract. That Daviel achieved wide acceptance of his method in the absence of existing ocular surgical instruments, suitable sutures, asepsis, or anesthesia makes this achievement all the more remarkable. His prominence and success gained in mastering this new and

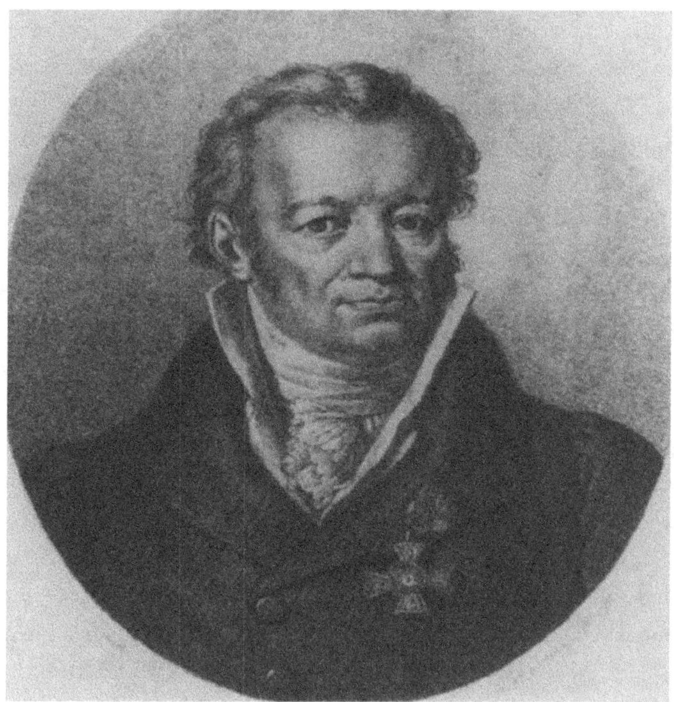

Fig. 11. Georg Joseph Beer (1763-1821) of Vienna, founder of an early European program training eye surgeons.
Source: Mark H. Georg Joseph Beer and Glaucoma. In: Leffler CT, ed. The History of Glaucoma. Wayenborgh. 2020:229-238.

difficult technique led others to follow his example, and ultimately caused the leading medical centers on the European continent to offer specialized training for eye surgeons. The first to do so was Austria, where Empress Maria Theresa appointed Joseph Beer to the first chair of ophthalmology in Vienna (Fig. 11). Major institutions throughout Europe followed their lead, marking the start of "modern ophthalmology."

References

1. Duchéne R, Contrucci J. Marseille: 2600 Ans D'histoire. Paris: Fayard; 1998.

2. Grangier R. Marseille and Jacques Daviel. *Hist Sci Medicales.* 2011;45(1):57-62.

3. Hildreth HR. Daviel: modern surgeon. *Am J Ophthalmol.* 1953;36(8):1071-1074. doi:10.1016/0002-9394(53)91888-1.

4. Chevalier JT. England's early oculist: pretender or pioneer? Parallel Press. 2014, November. https://www.library.wisc.edu/parallelpress/pp-catalog/additional-titles/chevalier-john-taylor-englandsearly-oculist-pretender-or-pioneer/. Accessed 2 October 2016.

5. Wallace W. *Boston Med Surg J.* 1844;30. Boston: Clapp D Jr.; https://books.google.com/books/about/The_Boston_Medical_and_Surgical_Journal.html?id=wE8sAAAAYAAJ. Accessed 3 October 2016.

6. Weiner DB. An eighteenth-century battle for priority: Jacques Daviel (1693-1762) and the extraction of cataracts. *J Hist Med Allied Sci.* 1986;41(2):129-155. doi:10.1093/jhmas/41.2.129.

7. Granit R. The grand theme of Stephen Polyak. *Science* 1955;122(3158):64. doi:10.1126/science.122.3158.64.

8. Polyak S, Kluver H, eds. *Vertebrate visual system*. Alibris Books. http://www.alibris.com/Vertebrate-Visual-System-Stephen-Polyak/book/7023551. Accessed 2 October 2016.

9. Duke-Elder S, Wybar K. *The anatomy of the visual system*. London: Kimpton; 1961.

10. Rucker CW. Cataract: a historical perspective. *Investig Ophthalmol.* 1965;4:377-383.

11. Peyronie F de La. Mémoires de L' Academie Royale de Chirurgie. Academie Royale de Chirurgie; 1753.

12. Villard C, Boissonnot M, Risse JF, et al. Ocular complication caused by fulguration. Discussion apropos of 2 simultaneous cases. *Bull Soc Ophtalmol Fr.* 1985;85(10):1027-1028. 1031-1034.

13. Mery J. Des Mouvements de l'Iris et par Occasion de la Partie Principale de l'Organe de la Vue. *Mém L'Académie R Sci Pour L'Année.* 1704:261-271.

14. Hubbell AA. Jacques Daviel and the beginnings of the modem operation of extraction of cataract: an address commemorative of the third semi-centennial anniversary of the publication of the first description of the operation. *J Am Med Assoc.* 1902;XXXIX(4):177. doi:10.1001/jama.1902.52480300001001a.

15. Shastid TH. Daviel, Jacques. In: Wood CA (ed.). *The American Encyclopedia and Dictionary of Ophthalmology* (Vol. V). Chicago: Cleveland Press; 1914:3751-3777.

16. Daviel J. Lettre de M. Daviel, Conseiller, Chirurgien ordinaire du Roi en Survivance & par quartier, à M. de Joyeuse, Docteur en Medecine de l'Université de Montpellier, Aggregé au Collége des Medecins de Marseille, & Médecin des Hôpitaux des Galéres. Paris: Mercure de France; September 1748:198-221.

17. Daviel J. Sur une Nouvelle Methode de Guérir la Cataracte par l'Extraction du Crystalllin. Mémoires de l'Académie Royale de Chirurgie, T. II, Paris; 1753:337-352.

18. Daviel JA, Pearce WG (trans.). On a new method to cure cataract by extraction of the lens by Jacques Daviel, translated by W. G. Pearce. *Brit J Ophthalmol.* July 1967;51(7):449-458.

19. Pouliquen Y. Un oculiste au siècle des lumières. Paris: Odile Jacob; 1999:182-183.

3. Aspiration of Cataract in 1815 in Philadelphia by Philip Syng Physick[1]

Christopher T. Leffler, MD, MPH[2]
Charles E. Letocha, MD[3]
Kasey Pierson, MD[2]
Stephen G. Schwartz, MD, MBA[4]

Introduction

Cataract extraction by suction through a narrow tube might have been attempted from time to time in the medieval Arabic period, and possibly even in antiquity.[1–5] According to standard accounts, the actual practice of cataract aspiration was reintroduced into the West by Stanislas Laugier of France in 1847.[1,4] However, we have uncovered an earlier 19th-century practitioner of cataract aspiration.

Account of a Patient with Cataracts in 1815

In 1815, 39-year-old attorney Francis B. Shaw (c. 1776-1832)[6] reported that he had been "deprived of sight by cataract" for over 2 years and forced to abandon his law practice, until surgeon Philip Syng Physick of Philadelphia successfully aspirated the cataract[7,8] (Figs. 1 and 2). Initially, surgeon John Syng Dorsey, the nephew of Physick, had operated on Shaw 3 times by the method of division.[7] This method, which enjoyed widespread popularity during this period, involved breaking up the cataract with a needle, with the intent that the remnants would be absorbed over a period of months.[9] Dorsey described his technique: After dilating the pupil with *Datura stramonium* (thorn apple, jimson weed), he introduced through the cornea a needle with which "the capsule and lens are to be torn in pieces: fragments of the lens can often be pushed forward into the anterior chamber of the eye, where they speedily dissolve."[10]

When this technique failed, Shaw proposed "drawing away the cataract and completely emptying the capsule of the lens."[7] Despite his poor vision, he designed the instruments, which he called "tubes and cannula points,"[11] and which were constructed by "an ingenious artist" under Shaw's direction.[7]

1 Partially supported by NIH Center Core Grant P30EY014801 and by an Unrestricted Grant from Research to Prevent Blindness to the University of Miami.

2 Department of Ophthalmology, Virginia Commonwealth University, Richmond, Virginia.

3 York, Pennsylvania.

4 Department of Ophthalmology, Bascom Palmer Eye Institute, University of Miami Miller School of Medicine, Naples, Florida.

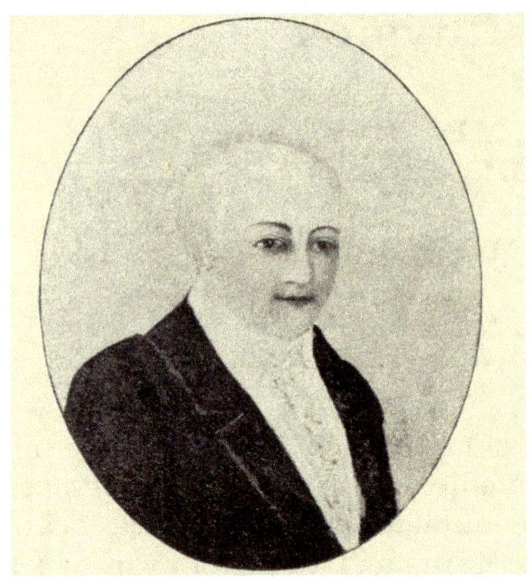

Fig. 1. Francis B. Shaw (c. 1776–1832).[6]

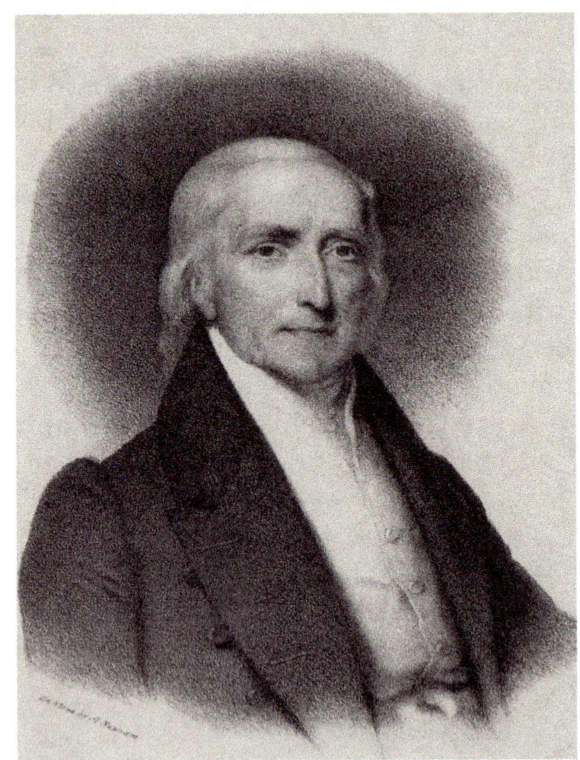

Fig. 2. Philip Syng Physick (1768–1837) of Philadelphia.

Shaw experimented with "different substances, as similar as possible to that of the cataract."[7] Using this method, Physick "completely removed every vestige of the Cataract, and the patient was once more restored to sight..."[7] Shaw was the first patient operated with this method[12] and was able to resume the practice of law within 3 months.[13]

That summer, Shaw obtained a federal patent for the system[12] for "Cataract, removing, by tubes."[14] Advantages included the ability to operate on cataracts at early stages before hardening or maturation and the fact that the lens capsule "is instantaneously fitted with a portion of the vitreous [sic] humor, and thereby its natural convexity preserved."[12] Of course, the refractive index of vitreous is too low to replace the lens. Still, Shaw might have imagined that postlensectomy ocular refractive function could be maintained with proper intracapsular contents, just as we do today with intraocular lenses. However, the state of Pennsylvania declined to purchase the patent rights in early 1816, because the method had only been used on two patients.[11]

Shaw had a financial interest in the matter, was not a surgeon, and did not describe the technique in detail. Therefore, it has been difficult to know how much credibility to give his account. Previously, historians have found no evidence from within the medical community to confirm that Physick aspirated cataracts.

Account of Surgeon Samuel White

On June 8, 1815, surgeon Samuel White (1777-1845), of Hudson, New York,[15] wrote to a fellow eye surgeon that he had "just returned from a tour" through hospitals in New York and Philadelphia (Fig. 3):

> I have also procured from Doct Physick his new invented Tubular instrument for extracting by suction the diseased lens when fluid. Shaw as was noticed in the papers, is not entitled to any credit for the construction. The operation is performed by Doct Physick by introducing a crow Lancet obliquely down thro' the cornea to the pupil, dipping the point so as to break the capsule, a curved silver tube is then introduced through the opening with the mouth of the tube on the back point, so as to be in contact with the lens, the operator then draws in the lens by suction and

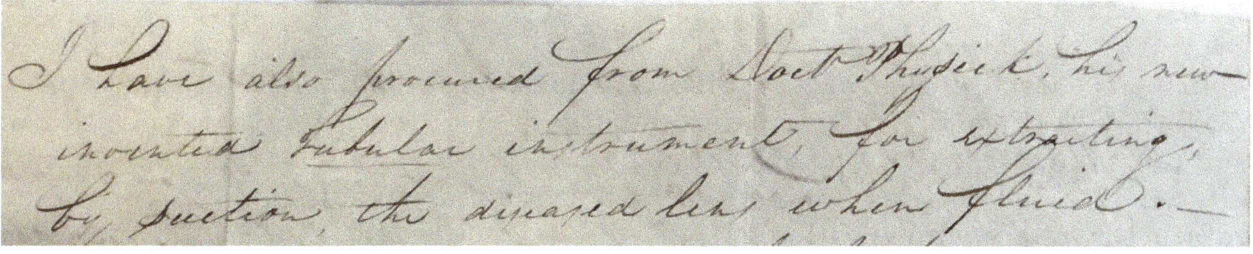

Fig. 3. Letter of surgeon Samuel White, dated June 8, 1815, describing cataract extraction by suction.[16]

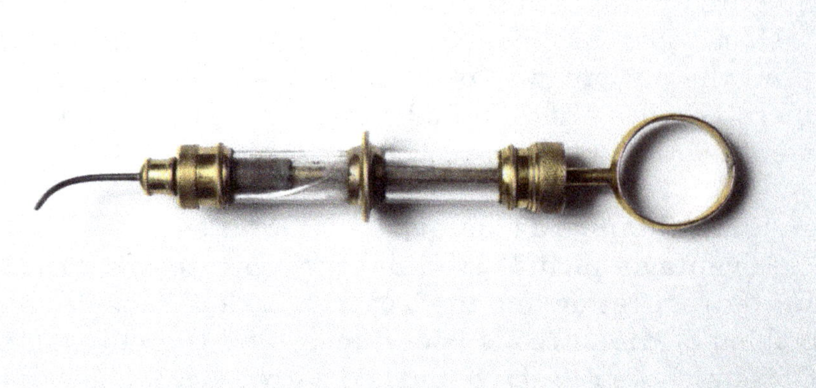

Fig. 4. Cannula attached to a syringe, from the cataract surgery instruments attributed to Philip Syng Physick, displayed at the Physick House in Philadelphia. (Courtesy of the College of Physicians of Philadelphia.)

withdraws the instrument from the eye. Doctor P. thinks this instrument may be improved to great advantage in cases of milky or fluid cataract—effecting in a few moments what otherwise might require months by absorption.[16]

Evidence from Philadelphia

In 1816, Dorsey wrote: "…Dr. Physick has successfully performed the ancient operation of sucking out a cataract by a small tube introduced through a puncture in the cornea. The operation is, however, attended with difficulties which will necessarily prevent its general adoption…"[10]

A set of cataract instruments attributed to Physick contains just one instrument resembling a "tube": a syringe that attaches to either a curved or straight cannula.[17] This instrument would appear suitable for cataract aspiration (Fig. 4). The University of Pennsylvania faculty did use syringes during this period,[18] specifically for aspiration of bodily fluids.[19] Thus, it appears Physick's method might have been more advanced than the oral suction technique used by Ammar.

Postscript

Fourteen years after the surgery, Shaw's vision was still sufficient for him to practice law.[20] In the mid-1800s, Laugier and others in Europe practiced aspiration of suitable cataracts.[1,4] Cataract aspiration became the dominant extraction technique after 1967, when Charles Kelman reported preliminary results in breaking up the cataract by phacoemulsification.[21]

References

1. Pérez-Cambrodí RJ, Ascaso FJ, Diab F, et al. Hollow needle cataract aspiration in antiquity. *Acta Ophthalmol.* 2015;93(8):782-784.

2. 'Ammār ibn 'Alī Mawṣilī, Meyerhof M. *Las Operaciones de catarata de 'Ammar ibn 'Ali al-Mawsili.* Barcelona, Spain: Laboratories del Norte de Espana; 1937:35-57.

3. Savage-Smith E. The practice of surgery in Islamic lands: myth and reality. Soc Hist Med. 2000 Aug;13(2):307-321.

4. Hirschberg J, Blodi FC. *The History of Ophthalmology. Vol. 2. The Middle Ages; The Sixteenth and Seventeenth Centuries.* Bonn, Germany: Wayenborgh Publishing; 1985:231-241.

5. Koch HR, Koch KR. Borri, the Prophet, on the "Restitutio Humorum" and on lens aspiration in the 17th century. *Proceedings of the Cogan Ophthalmic History Society.* New York, New York; 2015:246-262.

6. Davis WW. *History of Doylestown, Old and New.* Doylestown, Pennsylvania: Intelligencer Print; 1905:31-80.

7. Shaw FB. From the Philadelphia Daily Advertiser: Interesting Surgical Operation. *Commercial Advertiser.* April 3, 1815. New York, New York; XVIII(7063):2.

8. Letocha CE, Albert DM. 1815 Version of phacoemulsification? *Arch Ophthalmol.* 2010;128(1):19.

9. Leffler CT, Wainsztein RD. The first cataract surgeons in Latin America: 1611-1830. *Clin Ophthalmol.* 2016;10:679-694.

10. Cooper S, Dorsey JS, ed. *A Dictionary of Practical Surgery.* Vol. 1. Philadelphia: Kite; 1816:290.

11. No author listed. *Journal of the Twenty Sixth House of Representatives of the Commonwealth of Pennsylvania,* Vol. 26. Harrisburg: Peacock; January 31, 1816:204-296.

12. Shaw FB. The undersigned informs the public that he has obtained from the Department of State a patent. *Baltimore Patriot,* Vol VI(830). Baltimore; August 24, 1815:3.

13. Shaw FB. Francis B. Shaw … has resumed the practice of the law. *Pennsylvania Correspondent, and Farmers' Advertiser.* Doylestown, Pennsylvania; June 26, 1815: 3.

14. Burke E. *List of Patents for Inventions and Designs: Issued by the United States, from 1790 to 1847.* Washington: Gideon; 1847: 341.

15. Obituary Notice. *New York Journal of Medicine and the Collateral Sciences,* Vol. 4. New York: Langley; May 1845: 425-426.

16. White S. Letter from Samuel White to Mason Fitch Cogswell. *Mason Fitch Cogswell Papers.* General Collection, Beinecke Rare Book and Manuscript Library, Yale University. June 8, 1815; Series 1, Box 3, Folder 89.

17. Albert DM, Scheie HG. A history of ophthalmology at the University of Pennsylvania. Springfield, Illinois: Thomas; 1965: 11.

18. Dorsey JS. *Elements of surgery; for the use of students. Vol. 1.* Philadelphia: E. Parker; 1813: 297.

19. Dorsey JS. *Elements of surgery; for the use of students. Vol. 2.* Philadelphia: E. Parker; 1813: 149-408.

20. No author listed. Appointment by the Attorney General. Francis B. Shaw to be deputy attorney general for Bucks county. *Philadelphia Inquirer.* Philadelphia, Pennsylvania. July 23, 1829: 2.

21. Kelman CD. Phaco-emulsification and aspiration: A new technique of cataract removal: A preliminary report. *Am J Ophthalmol.* 1967;64(1):23-25.

A *New History of Cataract Surgery* consists of:

* Chapters origination from: *The History of Ophthalmology – The Monographs 15: The History of Glaucoma*